Meningiomas

Editors

GABRIEL ZADA
RANDY L. JENSEN

NEUROSURGERY
CLINICS OF NORTH AMERICA

www.neurosurgery.theclinics.com

Consulting Editors
RUSSELL LONSER
DANIEL K. RESNICK

April 2016 • Volume 27 • Number 2

ELSEVIER

1600 John F. Kennedy Boulevard • Suite 1800 • Philadelphia, Pennsylvania, 19103-2899

http://www.theclinics.com

NEUROSURGERY CLINICS OF NORTH AMERICA Volume 27, Number 2
April 2016 ISSN 1042-3680, ISBN-13: 978-0-323-44389-0

Editor: Jennifer Flynn-Briggs
Developmental Editor: Colleen Viola

Neurosurgery Clinics of North America (ISSN 1042-3680) is published quarterly by Elsevier Inc., 360 Park Avenue South, New York, NY 10010-1710. Months of issue are January, April, July, and October. Business and Editorial Offices: 1600 John F. Kennedy Blvd., Suite 1800, Philadelphia, PA 19103-2899. Customer Service Office: 11830 Westline Industrial Drive, St. Louis, MO 63146. Periodicals postage paid at New York, NY, and additional mailing offices. Subscription prices are $385.00 per year (US individuals), $639.00 per year (US institutions), $415.00 per year (Canadian individuals), $794.00 per year (Canadian institutions), $495.00 per year (international individuals), $794.00 per year (international institutions), $100.00 per year (US students), and $255.00 per year (international and Canadian students). International air speed delivery is included in all *Clinics* subscription prices. All prices are subject to change without notice. **POSTMASTER:** Send address changes to *Neurosurgery Clinics of North America*, Elsevier Periodicals Customer Service, 11830 Westline Industrial Drive, St. Louis, MO 63146. **Customer Service: 1-800-654-2452 (US and Canada). From outside the US and Canada, call: 1-314-453-7041. Fax: 1-314-453-5170. E-mail: JournalsCustomerService-usa@elsevier.com (for print support) and journalsonlinesupport-usa@elsevier.com (for online support).**

Reprints. For copies of 100 or more, of articles in this publication, please contact the Commercial Reprints Department, Elsevier Inc., 360 Park Avenue South, New York, NY 10010-1710. Tel. 212-633-3874; Fax: 212-633-3820; E-mail: reprints@elsevier.com.

Neurosurgery Clinics of North America is covered in *MEDLINE/PubMed (Index Medicus), EMBASE/Excerpta Medica, and Current Contents/Clinical Medicine (CC/CM).*

Contributors

CONSULTING EDITORS

RUSSELL LONSER, MD
Professor and Chair, Department of
Neurological Surgery, The Ohio State
University Wexner Medical Center, Columbus,
Ohio

DANIEL K. RESNICK, MD, MS
Professor and Vice Chairman, Program
Director, Department of Neurosurgery,
University of Wisconsin School of
Medicine and Public Health, Madison,
Wisconsin

EDITORS

GABRIEL ZADA, MD, MS
Assistant Clinical Professor of Neurosurgery,
Otolaryngology, and Medicine, Co-Director,
USC Pituitary Center; Co-Director, USC
Radiosurgery Center, Neuro-Oncology and
Endoscopic Pituitary/Skull Base Program,
Keck School of Medicine of USC, Los Angeles,
California

RANDY L. JENSEN, MD, PhD
Professor, Departments of Neurosurgery,
Oncological Sciences and Radiation Oncology,
Huntsman Cancer Institute, University of Utah,
Salt Lake City, Utah

AUTHORS

PANKAJ K. AGARWALLA, MD
Department of Cancer Biology,
Dana-Farber Cancer Institute,
Harvard Medical School, Boston,
Massachusetts

NATALIE BARNETTE, BS
Department of Neurological Surgery,
University of California Los Angeles,
Los Angeles, California

RAMEEN BEROUKHIM, MD, PhD
Department of Cancer Biology,
Dana-Farber Cancer Institute,
Harvard Medical School, Boston,
Massachusetts

NIKHILESH S. BHATT, BS
Department of Neurological Surgery,
University of California Los Angeles,
Los Angeles, California

WENYA LINDA BI, MD, PhD
Department of Neurosurgery, Brigham and
Women's Hospital; Department of Cancer
Biology, Dana-Farber Cancer Institute,
Harvard Medical School, Boston,
Massachusetts

OREST B. BOYKO, MD, PhD
Department of Radiology, Keck School of
Medicine, University of Southern California,
Los Angeles, California

SIMON BUTTRICK, MD
Resident, Department of Neurosurgery,
University of Miami, Coral Gables,
Florida

STEVEN Y. CEN, PhD
Department of Radiology, Keck School of
Medicine, University of Southern California,
Los Angeles, California

THOMAS C. CHEN, MD, PhD
Professor, Neurosurgery and Pathology, University of Southern California, Los Angeles, California

ADAM COHEN, MD
Assistant Professor, Department of Oncological Sciences, Huntsman Cancer Institute, University of Utah, Salt Lake City, Utah

OR COHEN-INBAR, MD, PhD
Department of Neurological Surgery, University of Virginia Health Sciences Center, Charlottesville, Virginia

HOWARD COLMAN, MD, PhD
Professor, Departments of Neurosurgery and Oncological Sciences, Huntsman Cancer Institute, University of Utah, Salt Lake City, Utah

FRANCESCO D'AMORE, MD
Department of Radiology, Keck School of Medicine, University of Southern California, Los Angeles, California

IAN F. DUNN, MD, FAANS, FACS
Department of Neurosurgery, Brigham and Women's Hospital, Harvard Medical School, Boston, Massachusetts

SVEN OLIVER EICKER, MD
Senior Staff Members, Department of Neurosurgery, University Medical Center Hamburg Eppendorf, Hamburg, Germany

PEDRAM EMAMI, MD
Senior Staff Members, Department of Neurosurgery, University Medical Center Hamburg Eppendorf, Hamburg, Germany

JOHN R. GAUGHEN Jr, MD
Department of Radiology and Medical Imaging, University of Virginia Health System, Charlottesville, Virginia

QUINTON GOPEN, MD
Department of Otolaryngology - Head & Neck Surgery, University of California Los Angeles, Los Angeles, California

JIAN GUAN, MD
Department of Neurosurgery, Clinical Neurosciences Center, University of Utah, Salt Lake City, Utah

DARRYL H. HWANG, PhD
Department of Radiology, Keck School of Medicine, University of Southern California, Los Angeles, California

MICHAEL E. IVAN, MD, MBS
Assistant Professor; Chief of Service, Cranial and Neuro-oncology, Department of Neurosurgery, Lois Pope Life Center, Co-Director of Neurosurgery, JSCH, University of Miami, Miami, Florida

ROBERT F. JAMES, MD
Department of Neurosurgery, University of Louisville School of Medicine, Louisville, Kentucky

RANDY L. JENSEN, MD, PhD
Professor, Departments of Neurosurgery, Oncological Sciences and Radiation Oncology, Huntsman Cancer Institute, University of Utah, Salt Lake City, Utah

MICHAEL KARSY, MD, PhD
Department of Neurosurgery, Clinical Neurosciences Center, University of Utah, Salt Lake City, Utah

PAUL E. KIM, MD
Department of Radiology, Keck School of Medicine, University of Southern California, Los Angeles, California

KEVIN S. KING, MD
Department of Radiology, Keck School of Medicine, University of Southern California, Los Angeles, California

RICARDO J. KOMOTAR, MD
Department of Neurosurgery, Co-Director of Neurooncology, Sylvester Comprehensive Cancer Center, University of Miami Health Clinics; Assistant Professor; Director of Neurooncology, University of Miami Hospital, University of Miami, Miami, Florida

DANIEL R. KRAMER, MD
Department of Neurosurgery, University of Southern California Keck School of Medicine, Los Angeles, California

MENG LAW, MD
Department of Radiology, Keck School of Medicine, University of Southern California, Los Angeles, California

CHENG-CHIA LEE, MD
Neurological Institute, Taipei Veteran General
Hospital, National Yang-Ming University,
Taipei, Taiwan

SEUNG JAMES LEE, BS
Department of Neurological Surgery, University
of California Los Angeles, Los Angeles,
California

ALEXANDER LERNER, MD
Department of Radiology, Keck School of
Medicine, University of Southern California,
Los Angeles, California

CHIA-SHANG J. LIU, MD, PhD
Department of Radiology, Keck School of
Medicine, University of Southern California,
Los Angeles, California

JOSHUA W. LUCAS, MD
Department of Neurosurgery, Keck School of
Medicine at USC, Los Angeles, California

WILLIAM J. MACK, MD
Department of Neurosurgery, University of
Southern California Keck School of Medicine,
Los Angeles, California

LACEY B. MARTIN, MD
Department of Neurosurgery, University of
Oklahoma School of Medicine, Norman,
Oklahoma

JAKOB MATSCHKE, MD
Senior Staff Members, Department of
Neuropathology, University Medical Center
Hamburg Eppendorf, Hamburg, Germany

YU MEI, MD, PhD
Department of Neurosurgery, Brigham and
Women's Hospital, Harvard Medical School,
Boston, Massachusetts

MALTE MOHME, MD
Resident, Department of Neurosurgery,
University Medical Center Hamburg
Eppendorf, Hamburg, Germany

PAUL S. PAGE, BS
Department of Neurosurgery, University of
Louisville School of Medicine, Louisville,
Kentucky

PANAYIOTIS E. PELARGOS, MS
Department of Neurological Surgery,
University of California Los Angeles,
Los Angeles, California

VIJAY M. RAVINDRA, MD, MSPH
Resident, Department of Neurosurgery,
Clinical Neurosciences Center, University of
Utah, Salt Lake City, Utah

JAN REGELSBERGER, MD
Senior Staff Members, Department of
Neurosurgery, University Medical Center
Hamburg Eppendorf, Hamburg, Germany

MEIC H. SCHMIDT, MD, MBA
Professor, Department of Neurosurgery,
Clinical Neurosciences Center, University of
Utah, Salt Lake City, Utah

ASHISH H. SHAH, MD
Resident, Department of Neurosurgery,
University of Miami, Coral Gables, Florida

JASON P. SHEEHAN, MD, PhD
Department of Neurological Surgery,
University of Virginia Health Sciences Center,
Charlottesville, Virginia

MARK S. SHIROISHI, MD
Department of Radiology, Keck School of
Medicine, University of Southern California,
Los Angeles, California

MARKO SPASIC, MD
Department of Neurological Surgery,
University of California Los Angeles,
Los Angeles, California

BENITA TAMRAZI, MD
Pediatric Neuroradiology; Department of
Radiology, Children's Hospital Los Angeles;
Keck School of Medicine, University of
Southern California, Los Angeles, California

NOLAN UNG, BS
Department of Neurological Surgery,
University of California Los Angeles,
Los Angeles, California

MANFRED WESTPHAL, MD
Chairman, Department of Neurosurgery,
University Medical Center Hamburg
Eppendorf, Hamburg, Germany

ISAAC YANG, MD
Attending Neurosurgeon, Assistant Professor, Department of Neurosurgery, Director of Medical Student Education, Jonsson Comprehensive Cancer Center, David Geffen School of Medicine at UCLA; Department of Neurological Surgery, University of California Los Angeles, Los Angeles, California

GABRIEL ZADA, MD, MS
Assistant Clinical Professor of Neurosurgery, Otolaryngology, and Medicine, Co-Director, USC Pituitary Center; Co-Director, USC Radiosurgery Center, Neuro-Oncology and Endoscopic Pituitary/Skull Base Program, Keck School of Medicine of USC, Los Angeles, California

Contents

> Although typically not necessary for the diagnosis of intracranial meningiomas, advanced imaging techniques, including perfusion and diffusion imaging, spectroscopy, and nuclear medicine imaging, can help confirm the diagnosis of intracranial meningiomas, especially for meningiomas that do not exhibit the typical anatomic imaging findings. Advanced imaging techniques also have the potential to be able to differentiate between the subtypes of meningiomas, predict clinical aggressiveness of the tumor, and better characterize response to treatment. Although no advanced imaging technique has been able to definitively subclassify meningiomas, current results are encouraging and may be helpful in surgical planning.

> This article provides an overview of the neuroimaging literature focused on preoperative prediction of meningioma consistency. A validated, noninvasive neuroimaging method to predict tumor consistency can provide valuable information regarding neurosurgical planning and patient counseling. Most of the neuroimaging literature indicates conventional MRI using T2-weighted imaging may be helpful to predict meningioma consistency; however, further rigorous validation is necessary. Much less is known about advanced MRI techniques, such as diffusion MRI, MR elastography (MRE), and MR spectroscopy. Of these methods, MRE and diffusion tensor imaging appear particularly promising.

> Endovascular embolization is a frequently-used adjunct to operative resection of meningiomas. Embolization may decrease intraoperative blood loss, operative time, and surgical difficulty associated with resection. The specific clinical applications of this treatment have not been defined clearly. Procedural indications, preferred embolic agent, and latency until tumor resection all differ across operators. It is clear that strategic patient selection, comprehensive anatomic understanding, and sound operative technique are critical to the success of the embolization procedure. This article reviews the management and technical considerations associated with preoperative meningioma embolization.

Meningiomas are the most common primary intracranial neoplasms in adults. Despite their prevalence, their biologic underpinnings remain incompletely described. The recent application of unbiased next-generation sequencing and epigenomic approaches has implicated a new array of candidate biomarkers and oncogenic drivers. These insights may serve to craft a molecular taxonomy for meningiomas and highlight putative therapeutic targets in an era of biology-informed precision medicine.

Secretory meningiomas (SM) represent a rare variant of the most common benign intracranial brain tumor. Defined by the histologic appearance of eosinophilic glandular formations and periodic-acidic Schiff–positive pseudopsammoma bodies, SM are characterized by unique molecular alterations, a disproportional occurrence of reactive peritumoral brain edema, and a clinical course that demands for increased awareness for perioperative complications. The frequent presence of extensive peritumoral edema has become a hallmark of SM and can be associated with life-threatening complications. The exact pathophysiology of edema formation in SM is still unknown.

Primary intraosseous meningiomas are a subtype of primary extradural meningiomas. They represent approximately two-thirds of extradural meningiomas and fewer than 2% of meningiomas overall. These tumors originate within the bones of the skull and can have a clinical presentation and radiographic differential diagnosis different from those for intradural meningiomas. Primary intraosseous meningiomas are classified based on location and histopathologic characteristics. Treatment is primarily surgical resection with wide margins if possible. Sparse literature exists regarding the use of adjuvant therapies. The literature regarding primary intraosseous meningiomas consists primarily of clinical case reports and case series. This literature is reviewed and summarized in this article.

 Video content accompanies this article at http://www.neurosurgery.theclinics.com

Spinal meningiomas are the most common spinal tumors encountered in adults, and account for 6.5% of all craniospinal tumors. The treatment for these lesions is primarily surgical, but emerging modalities may include chemotherapy and radiosurgery. In this article, the current management of spinal meningiomas and the body of literature surrounding conventional treatment are reviewed and discussed.

The resection of anterior skull base meningiomas has traditionally been performed via pterional or unilateral/bilateral subfrontal craniotomies. The supraorbital keyhole approach and the endoscopic endonasal approach, techniques in which the endoscope is used to aid visualization, were developed to provide alternative, less-invasive approaches to aid the resection of these tumors. The individual characteristics of each tumor, such as location and size, are the main determinants guiding the choice of approach. In this article, the advantages and disadvantages of each approach are discussed, along with complications specific to each technique. Furthermore, a detailed procedural description of each surgical approach is described.

Meningiomas are among the most common intracranial tumors in adults. The mainstay of treatment has been extirpation. Stereotactic radiosurgery (SRS) is an important option in the management of inaccessible, recurrent, or residual benign meningiomas. Image guidance and a steep dose fall off are critical features. SRS offers durable tumor control for grade I meningiomas with a low incidence of complications or neurologic deficits. Neurologic function is generally preserved or improved. Complications are relatively rare. For many, the risk to benefit ratio seems favorable compared with treatment alternatives. We present a short review of the literature on SRS for intracranial meningiomas.

The number of patient imaging studies has increased because of precautious physicians ordering scans when a vague symptom is presented; subsequently, the number of incidental meningiomas detected has increased as well. These brain tumors do not present with related symptoms and are usually small. MRI and computed tomographic scans most frequently capture incidental meningiomas. Incidental meningiomas are managed with observation, radiation, and surgical resection. Ultimately, a conservative approach is recommended, such as observing an incidental meningioma and then only radiating if the tumor displays growth, whereas a surgical approach is to be used only when proven necessary.

Meningiomas are the most prevalent primary tumor of central nervous system origin and, although most neoplasms are benign, a small proportion exemplifies an aggressive profile characterized by high recurrence rates, pleomorphic histology, and overall resistance to standard treatment. Standard initial therapy for malignant meningiomas includes maximal safe surgical resection followed by focal radiation in certain cases. The role for chemotherapy during recurrence of these aggressive

NEUROSURGERY CLINICS OF NORTH AMERICA

THE CLINICS ARE AVAILABLE ONLINE!
Access your subscription at:
www.theclinics.com

Preface
Meningiomas: An Update on Diagnostic and Therapeutic Approaches

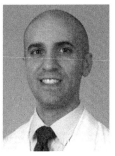 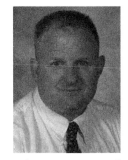

Gabriel Zada, MD, MS   Randy L. Jensen, MD, PhD
Editors

Advances in imaging, diagnostics, and therapeutics have improved the contemporary care of patients with meningiomas. In this issue, we examine emerging advanced neuroimaging techniques, including preoperative characteristics that may predict consistency of meningiomas. Endovascular techniques to reduce risk and improve surgical resection of meningiomas are also examined. New diagnostic modalities, including genomic and epigenomic biomarkers, are emerging to aid molecular classification and even potentially open new avenues of signal pathway blockade. Special meningioma subtypes, including secretory, spinal, and interosseous meningiomas, are discussed, with an emphasis on the unique nature of these tumors. Specialized treatment techniques, such as the minimally invasive, endoscopic, and noninvasive stereotactic radiosurgical methods, are outlined. Finally, management of incidental, atypical, and treatment-refractory meningiomas is explored and controversies outlined. It is hoped that these articles will provide cutting-edge information to improve the care of patients with meningiomas.

Gabriel Zada, MD, MS
USC Pituitary Center
USC Radiosurgery Center
Neuro-Oncology and Endoscopic Pituitary/
Skull Base Program
Keck School of Medicine of USC
1520 San Pablo Street #3800
Los Angeles, CA 90033, USA

Randy L. Jensen, MD, PhD
Huntsman Cancer Institute
University of Utah
5th Floor CNC
175 North Medical Drive
Salt Lake City, UT 84132, USA

E-mail addresses:
gzada@usc.edu (G. Zada)
Randy.jensen@hsc.utah.edu (R.L. Jensen)

Neurosurg Clin N Am 27 (2016) xiii
http://dx.doi.org/10.1016/j.nec.2016.02.001
1042-3680/16/$ – see front matter © 2016 Published by Elsevier Inc.

Advanced Imaging of Intracranial Meningiomas

 CrossMark

Benita Tamrazi, MD[a], Mark S. Shiroishi, MD[b], Chia-Shang J. Liu, MD, PhD[b],*

KEYWORDS

- Meningioma • Perfusion • Diffusion • Spectroscopy • MRI • CT • PET • SPECT

KEY POINTS

- Conventional anatomic imaging is typically adequate to distinguish intracranial meningiomas from other tumors, but advanced imaging techniques can help confirm the diagnosis in equivocal cases.
- Meningiomas demonstrate elevated cerebral blood flow/cerebral blood volume on perfusion imaging, with the perfusion characteristics helpful to distinguish it from other intracranial neoplasms, as well as potentially characterizing the subtype of meningioma.
- Different types of meningiomas have been shown to have differences in diffusivity, but more recent larger sample studies have not shown diffusion imaging as a reliable way of differentiating meningioma histopathologic types.
- Spectroscopy provides molecular information with regard to meningiomas and can potentially reflect genetic heterogeneity within a tumor and aid biopsy planning.
- Radionuclides that bind somatostatin receptors can be a sensitive and specific method of characterizing meningiomas.

BACKGROUND

Meningiomas arise from the arachnoid meningothelial cells. Intracranially, they are extra-axial masses that are typically T1 isointense to slightly hypointense and T2 hyperintense to cortex, demonstrating avid and often homogeneous postcontrast enhancement. Differentiating meningiomas from other intracranial masses typically involve identifying the extra-axial nature of the mass, with evidence of hyperostosis of the adjacent osseous structures, as well as presence of calcification within the mass helpful for confirming the diagnosis of meningioma. The imaging appearance of meningiomas on MRI is typically characteristic enough that routine imaging sequences of T1-weighted and T2-weighted sequences, as well as postcontrast T1-weighted sequences are sufficient in making the diagnosis.[1]

Differentiating different subtypes of typical meningiomas and distinguishing typical from atypical/malignant meningiomas may not be possible from the conventional MRI sequences, however. Also, distinguishing meningiomas from other dural-based extra-axial masses, such as in a patient with a known primary malignancy that has a finding of a dural-based extra-axial mass intracranially, would be difficult with conventional T1-weighted and T2-weighted sequences alone. Distinguishing cystic meningiomas from other rim-enhancing/necrotic neoplasms, such as glioblastoma multiforme, also can be difficult, especially when the mass is large and there is difficulty identifying whether or not the mass is intra-axial or extra-axial.[1]

Diffusion-weighted imaging/diffusion tensor imaging (DWI/DTI), perfusion imaging, and magnetic resonance spectroscopy (MRS) can add

Funding: M.S. Shiroishi supported in part by SC CTSI (NIH/NCRR/NCATS) Grant KL2TR000131, Toshiba American Medical Systems and is a consultant for Guerbet.
[a] Department of Radiology, Children's Hospital Los Angeles, 4650 Sunset Boulevard, Los Angeles, CA 90027, USA; [b] Department of Radiology, Keck School of Medicine, University of Southern California, 1500 San Pablo Street, Los Angeles, CA 90033, USA
* Corresponding author.
E-mail address: chia-shang.liu@med.usc.edu

Neurosurg Clin N Am 27 (2016) 137–143
http://dx.doi.org/10.1016/j.nec.2015.11.004
1042-3680/16/$ – see front matter © 2016 Elsevier Inc. All rights reserved.

additional information that can help refine the diagnostic considerations of a dural-based mass and has the potential to characterize the different subtypes of meningiomas. This article reviews the imaging findings of the techniques as they apply to meningiomas.

PERFUSION IMAGING

Although routine diagnostic MRI of the brain without and with intravenous contrast is typically able to diagnose a meningioma, it may sometimes be difficult to differentiate a mass as intra-axial or extra-axial in location because of the location or size of the mass. Magnetic resonance perfusion (MR perfusion) can potentially help differentiate a primary glial neoplastic process from an extra-axial mass. MR perfusion can be performed either with a dynamic susceptibility contrast (DSC) technique or a dynamic contrast enhancement (DCE) technique, both of which require the administration of intravenous gadolinium. The two techniques differ in the image acquisition sequence used, with DSC using an echo planar imaging technique and DCE using a gradient echo imaging technique. Both techniques require rapid administration of intravenous gadolinium in a quick bolus, with rapid imaging of the area of interest performed, typically approximately 40 volumes in a 2-minute to 5-minute period.[2–4]

DSC MR perfusion, the more typically used of the MR perfusion techniques, measures relative cerebral blood volume. Neoplastic processes typically have elevated relative cerebral blood volume compared with the contralateral white matter, and MR perfusion can identify masses with elevated relative cerebral blood volume. The time course of DSC MR perfusion also differs for primarily glial neoplastic processes as compared with intracranial metastases/extra-axial masses. The DSC signal time curve of a primary glial neoplastic process typically demonstrates greater than 50% return to baseline, whereas the DSC signal time curve for metastases/extra-axial masses typically demonstrates less than 50% return to baseline due to the increased breakdown in blood-brain barrier as well as the presence of dural-based blood supply for metastases/extra-axial masses.[5,6]

Fig. 1 illustrates the utility of MR perfusion in characterizing meningiomas. A patient from our institution with a history of multiple meningiomas and resection of a large right frontal meningioma in the past presented for follow-up imaging. On the postcontrast axial T1 sequence (see **Fig. 1**A), there was a left frontal dural-based homogeneously enhancing extra-axial mass compatible with a meningioma, along with a smaller meningioma along the falx. MR perfusion was performed (**Fig. 2**B), with a region of interest (ROI) placed on the normal, contralateral white matter (ROI #1, green) and another placed on the left frontal meningioma (ROI #2, purple). The contrast enhancement time curve of the left frontal meningioma (curve #2, purple) demonstrates elevated relative cerebral blood volume when compared with the contrast-enhancement time curve of the contralateral white matter

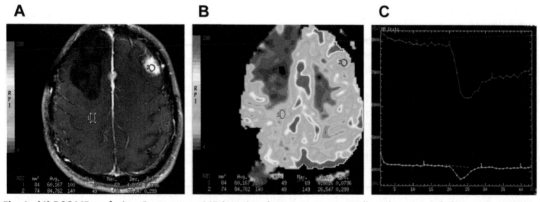

Fig. 1. (A) DSC MR perfusion. Postcontrast MR imaging demonstrates an avidly enhancing left frontal dural-based extra-axial mass. The patient had a right frontal meningioma that had been resected in the past, with an additional meningioma seen along the anterior falx. (B) Perfusion analysis is performed by placing an ROI on the enhancing mass in the perfusion sequence (ROI #2, *purple*) and comparing it with the contralateral white matter (ROI #1, *green*). (C) The time course of the perfusion curves demonstrates the left frontal mass to have a loss of signal from the susceptibility effect of the gadolinium contrast of a greater magnitude than the contralateral white matter, signifying elevated relative cerebral blood volume, with less than 50% return to baseline for the perfusion curve of the mass, characteristic of extra-axial, nonglial tumors such as meningiomas.

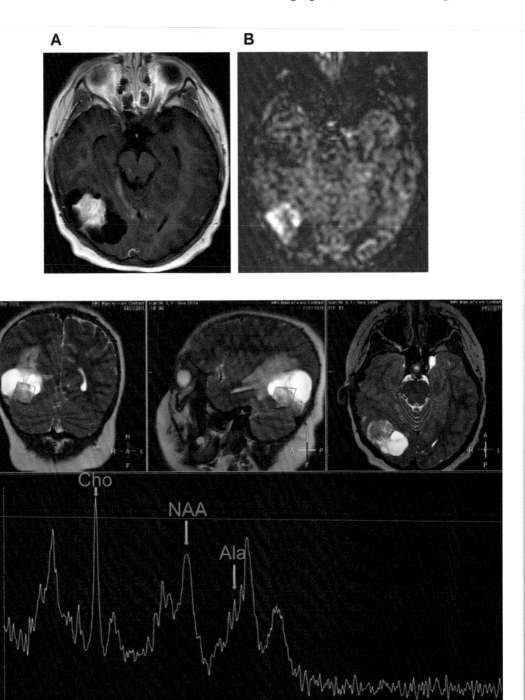

Fig. 2. (*A*) Postcontrast imaging demonstrates a large centrally enhancing right temporo-occipital mass with peripheral cystic components. It is difficult to definitively ascertain if the mass is extra-axial or intra-axial. (*B*) ASL demonstrates increased signal within the enhancing component of the mass, compatible with elevated cerebral blood flow, which can be seen in meningiomas. (*C*) MR spectroscopy demonstrates a prominent Ala peak at 1.48 ppm, elevated Cho peak at 3.2 ppm, and decreased NAA peak at 2.0 ppm. These findings are compatible with a meningioma. Elevated spectroscopic peaks are also seen at 3.8 ppm, which has also been reported to be elevated in meningiomas. Prominent lipid/lactate peak also is seen.

(curve #1, green), with the contrast-enhancement time curve of the meningioma demonstrating less than 50% return to baseline, which is the typical perfusion behavior of meningiomas as described in the literature (**Fig. 2**C).

MR perfusion also has been used to differentiate subtypes of meningiomas as well as differentiating typical from atypical meningiomas. Angiomatous meningiomas have been shown to have significantly higher tumoral relative cerebral blood volume compared with meningothelial, fibrous, or anaplastic meningiomas, and anaplastic meningiomas have higher peritumoral relative cerebral blood volume compared with the other types of meningiomas.[7] Peritumoral edema surrounding malignant meningiomas (World Health Organization [WHO] grade III) also has been shown to have increased relative cerebral blood volume compared with benign meningiomas (WHO grade I) via MR perfusion imaging.[8] The volume transfer constant, K^{trans}, which is a measurement of vascular permeability, for atypical meningiomas (WHO grade II) has been shown to be higher than that for typical (benign) meningiomas.[9]

MR perfusion also can be performed to evaluate the contributions of the blood supply to the meningioma. Intra-arterial injection of gadolinium via catheter selection of the internal and external carotid arteries, in combination with intraoperative MR perfusion, can differentiate which portions of the tumors are supplied by which arterial supply. MR perfusion also can be performed after the embolization to assess for residual perfusion to the treated meningioma.[10,11]

Arterial spin labeling (ASL) is an MRI technique in which a radiofrequency pulse is applied to the arteries proximal to the ROI in such a way that the protons in the inflowing blood have a detectable signal. Cerebral blood flow can therefore be calculated in the ROI as a function of increased amount of "tagged" blood that has flowed into the ROI. ASL does not require the use of intravenous gadolinium, and therefore has the advantage of being usable even in patients with impaired renal function who otherwise may not be able to receive intravenous gadolinium. ASL has been shown to be able to detect increased cerebral blood flow within meningiomas, with the technique also demonstrating statistically significant increased cerebral blood flow in angiomatous meningiomas compared with fibrous and meningothelial meningiomas[12] (see **Fig. 2**B).

Although not typically used to diagnose meningiomas, computed tomography (CT) perfusion, like ASL, can more conspicuously identify intracranial meningiomas due to the increased cerebral blood flow and cerebral blood volume within the meningiomas[13] (**Fig. 3**). Although the meningioma may be less distinct in a noncontrast head CT, blending into the adjacent brain parenchyma (see **Fig. 3**A), CT perfusion, performed due to suspicion of stroke in this case, demonstrates a left frontal mass with elevated cerebral blood volume (see **Fig. 3**B) as well as elevated cerebral blood flow (see **Fig. 3**C) when compared with the adjacent as well as contralateral brain parenchyma. A contrast-enhanced head CT also clearly delineates the left frontal meningioma from the brain parenchyma (see **Fig. 3**D).

CT perfusion also has been used to characterize the peritumoral edema around meningiomas, with decreased cerebral blood flow seen in the peritumoral edema, potentially reflective of ischemic tissue that may be salvageable after resection of the tumor.[14] The findings are similar to that from MR perfusion, which suggest that the decrease in relative cerebral blood volume may be a consequence of, rather than the cause of, the vasogenic edema, and that ischemic changes may be a secondary facultative phenomenon in the pathogenesis of meningioma-related brain edema.[15]

CT perfusion also has been used to differentiate meningiomas from hemangiopericytomas, extra-axial masses that are at times difficult to differentiate from meningiomas by conventional imaging features alone and clinically have more aggressive features and higher probability of recurrence and metastasis than meningiomas.[16] CT perfusion analysis has demonstrated that hemangiopericytomas have increased cerebral blood volume compared with benign meningiomas, with the permeability surface, a measure of microvascular permeability, also higher in hemangiopericytomas compared with benign meningiomas.[17]

Perfusion imaging of the brain also can be performed using radionuclides, specifically technetium-99m-d, 1-hexamethyipropyleneamine oxime (^{99m}Tc-d, 1-HMPAO). ^{99m}Tc-d, 1-HMPAO single-photon emission CT has been used to characterize intracranial tumors, and meningiomas have been shown to have significantly higher HMPAO uptake, corresponding to increased cerebral blood flow, compared with gliomas.[18]

DIFFUSION IMAGING

Diffusion MRI is an imaging technique that can measure the degree of mobility of water molecules within a biological tissue. By applying gradient fields in a specific way that refocuses the signal of the biological tissue in the MRI scanner except for the signal loss that occurs as a result of the Brownian motion of water, the

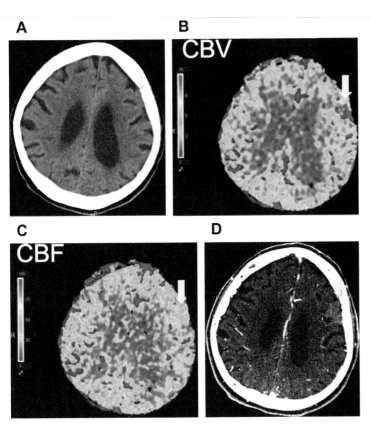

Fig. 3. Incidental finding of a meningioma. (*A*) Noncontrast head CT for a patient with stroke symptoms demonstrates a subtle left frontal extra-axial mass that is isoattenuating to brain parenchyma (*yellow arrow*). (*B*) CT perfusion demonstrates elevated cerebral blood volume (CBV) and (*C*) cerebral blood flow (CBF) within the left frontal mass (*yellow arrow*), which can be seen in a meningioma. (*D*) CT angiography of the head demonstrates the left frontal extra-axial mass (*yellow arrow*) with arterial phase enhancement, compatible with a meningioma.

magnitude of Brownian motion within the biological tissue can be measured, which can be a proxy of cellularity of the tissue, reflect evidence of injury in the context of cytotoxic edema, and elucidate orientation of macromolecular structures, such as white matter fiber tracts.[19] Measurements of apparent diffusion coefficients (ADCs) can be made with diffusion MRI, with decreased ADC reflective of decreased Brownian motion of water and therefore suggestive of increased cellularity or cytotoxic edema. Other parameters that can be measured on diffusion MRI include fractional anisotropy (FA), a measure of how directional the water motion in a given area is, with a higher FA indicative of increased directionality of water motion, and a lower FA indicative of more diffuse, random water motion.

The ability for diffusion MRI to characterize cellular tumors has led to research into the application of diffusion MRI to characterize different types of meningiomas. Early research demonstrated that lower ADC values are seen in atypical or malignant meningiomas compared with normal brain parenchyma or benign meningiomas with the exception of densely calcified or psammomatous meningiomas,[20] with a subsequent study with more subjects in both the atypical/malignant meningioma

as well as benign meningioma groups also demonstrating similar results.[21] A study using DTI, which assesses not only for diffusivity of the water molecules but also the directionality of diffusion, also demonstrated that atypical meningiomas have decreased ADC compared with benign meningiomas, and that benign meningiomas have a lower FA, or more spherical diffusivity, compared with atypical meningiomas.[22] More recent studies, with a much larger sample size compared with the earlier studies, did not find a statistically significant difference between the ADC values of atypical and benign meningiomas, nor were the ADC values statistically different for the various histologic subtypes of meningiomas.[23,24]

SPECTROSCOPY

MR spectroscopy has the ability to evaluate for the concentration of metabolites within a given ROI. Rather than detecting the resonance signal of protons (predominantly water) relative to spatial location after the application of a gradient pulse and assessing the morphology of a lesion of interest, the resonance signal of the protons from the different molecular groups within the lesion of interest, such as N-acetylaspartate (NAA), choline

(Cho), creatine (Cr), glutamine/glutamate (Glx), alanine (Ala), and lactate (Lac), can be detected. Identifying the chemical composition of the lesion of interest is not only useful for identifying metabolic abnormalities but can be helpful in identifying neoplastic processes as well.

Meningiomas have been shown to have elevated Cho and decreased NAA, which is also seen in many other neoplastic processes. There also is a decrease in Cr.[25] Prominent Ala is also seen in meningiomas, much more so than in other neoplastic processes and is considered a spectroscopic signature for meningiomas.[26]

The utility of MR spectroscopy in characterizing meningiomas is seen in a patient who presents with a large right parietotemporal cystic mass with a large centrally enhancing component (Fig. 2A). Diagnostic considerations based on conventional imaging for this mass include intra-axial masses such as a glioma as well as extra-axial masses such as a meningioma. ASL demonstrates increased signal within the mass, compatible with elevated cerebral blood flow (see Fig. 2B), which can be seen in both meningiomas and gliomas. MR spectroscopy of the mass demonstrates a prominent Ala peak, decreased NAA peak, and elevated Cho peak, however, confirming that the mass is indeed a meningioma (see Fig. 2C).

An elevated metabolite peak at 3.8 parts per million (ppm) also has been described in meningiomas, which is nearly absent in high-grade gliomas and intracranial metastasis in one study.[27] Ex vivo MRS evaluation of meningiomas with different genetic mutations also have demonstrated differences in the detected metabolites, with WHO grade I meningiomas having 1p, 14q, and/or 22q genetic mutations, mutations that have been shown to result in rapid recurrence of tumor, demonstrating decreased Ala concentrations compared with WHO grade I meningiomas without those genetic aberrations.[28] Ex vivo MRS evaluations have also attempted to characterize the various subtypes of meningiomas, demonstrating differences in macromolecular and lipid peaks in meningothelial, fibrous, and oncocytic subtypes of meningiomas.[29] The knowledge that heterogeneity of tumoral tissue may reflect underlying genetic heterogeneity, and that MRS can potentially characterize more clinically aggressive portions of tumors, have led to the use of MRS in neuronavigation for surgical biopsy.[30]

NUCLEAR MEDICINE

Nuclear medicine techniques to evaluate for increased perfusion of meningiomas have already been described in the section on perfusion imaging. Radionuclides also have been made to target somatostatin receptors, which are expressed in meningiomas. Indium-111–labeled octreotide, as well as technetium-99m–labeled depreotide, have been used with single-photon emission CT to image meningiomas,[31] with gallium-68–labeled DOTA-D-Phe1-Tyr3-octreotide, which has a high affinity for the somatostatin receptor subtype 2 (SSTR 2), used with PET to image meningiomas. The high tumor-to-background ratio, along with the advent of hybrid PET and MRI systems, allow for highly sensitive and specific diagnosis of intracranial meningiomas.[32]

SUMMARY

Although the diagnosis of intracranial meningioma often can be made with conventional anatomic imaging, advanced imaging techniques have the potential to not only confirm the presumptive anatomic imaging diagnosis of a meningioma, but they also have the potential to differentiate the histologic subtypes of meningiomas as well as predict the clinical aggressiveness of the tumor. Definitive subtyping of meningiomas is still not possible by imaging alone at this time, but continued advances in imaging technique will give the clinicians more information with regard to the meningioma before surgery.

REFERENCES

1. Buetow MP, Buetow PC, Smirniotopoulos JG. Typical, atypical, and misleading features in meningioma. Radiographics 1991;11(6):1087–106.
2. Shiroishi MS, Castellazzi G, Boxerman JL, et al. Principles of T2*-weighted dynamic susceptibility contrast MRI techniques in brain tumor imaging. J Magn Reson Imaging 2015;41:296–313.
3. Shiroishi MS, Habibi M, Rajderkar D, et al. Perfusion and permeability MR imaging of gliomas. Technol Cancer Res Treat 2011;10(1):59–71.
4. Essig M, Shiroishi MS, Nguyen TB, et al. Perfusion MRI: the five most frequently asked technical questions. AJR Am J Roentgenol 2013;200:24–34.
5. Cha S, Knopp EA, Johnson G, et al. Intracranial mass lesions: dynamic contrast-enhanced susceptibility-weighted echo-planar perfusion MR imaging. Radiology 2002;223:11–29.
6. Hakyemez B, Yildirim N, Erdoğan C, et al. Meningiomas with conventional MRI findings resembling intraaxial tumors: can perfusion-weighted MRI be helpful in differentiation? Neuroradiology 2006;48: 695–702.
7. Zang H, Rödinger LA, Shen T, et al. Preoperative subtyping of meningiomas by perfusion MR imaging. Neuroradiology 2008;50:835–40.

8. Zang H, Rödinger LA, Shen T, et al. Perfusion MR imaging for differentiation of benign and malignant meningiomas. Neuroradiology 2008;50:525–30.

9. Yang S, Law M, Zagzag D, et al. Dynamic contrast-enhanced perfusion MR imaging measurements of endothelial permeability: differentiating between atypical and typical meningiomas. AJNR Am J Neuroradiol 2003;24:1554–9.

10. Saloner D, Uzelac A, Hetts S, et al. Modern meningioma imaging techniques. J Neurooncol 2010;99: 333–40.

11. Martin AJ, Cha S, Higashida RT, et al. Assessment of vasculature of meningiomas and the effects of embolization with intra-arterial MR perfusion imaging: a feasibility study. AJNR Am J Neuroradiol 2007;28:1771–7.

12. Kimura H, Takeuchi H, Koshimoto Y, et al. Perfusion imaging of meningiomas by using continuous arterial spin labeling: comparison with dynamic susceptibility-weighted contrast-enhanced MR images and histopathologic features. AJNR Am J Neuroradiol 2006;27:85–93.

13. Tamrazi B, Yuh E. Stroke mimics imaging atlas: pearls and pitfalls in interpretation of brain CT perfusion studies. Proc Am Soc Neuroradiol 2013;51: 736–7. Available online at: http://www.asnr.org/sites/default/files/proceedings/2013.pdf.

14. Sergides I, Hussain Z, Naik S, et al. Utilization of dynamic CT perfusion in the study of intracranial meningiomas and their surrounding tissue. Neurol Res 2009;31:84–9.

15. Bitzer M, Klose U, Geist-Barth B, et al. Alteration in diffusion and perfusion in the pathogenesis of peritumoral brain edema in meningiomas. Eur Radiol 2002;12:2062–76.

16. Sibtain NA, Butt S, Connor SEJ. Imaging features of central nervous system haemangiopericytomas. Eur Radiol 2007;17:1685–93.

17. Ren G, Chen S, Wang Y, et al. Quantitative evaluation of benign meningioma and hemangiopericytoma with peritumoral brain edema by 64-slice CT perfusion imaging. Chin Med J 2010;123(15): 2038–44.

18. Suess E, Malessa S, Ungersböck K, et al. Technetium-99m-d,1-hexamethylpropyleneamine oxime (HMPAO) uptake and glutathione content in brain tumors. J Nucl Med 1991;32(9):1675–81.

19. Schaefer PW, Grant PE, Gonzalez RG. Diffusion-weighted MR imaging of the brain. Radiology 2000;217:331–45.

20. Filippi CG, Edgar MA, Uluğ AM, et al. Appearance of meningiomas on diffusion-weighted images: correlating diffusion constants with histopathologic findings. AJNR Am J Neuroradiol 2001;22:65–72.

21. Nagar VA, Ye JR, Ng WH, et al. Diffusion-weighted MR imaging: diagnosing atypical or malignant meningiomas and detecting tumor dedifferentiation. AJNR Am J Neuroradiol 2008;29:1147–52.

22. Toh CH, Castillo M, Wong AM, et al. Differentiation between classic and atypical meningiomas with use of diffusion tensor imaging. AJNR Am J Neuroradiol 2008;29:1630–5.

23. Santelli L, Ramondo G, Della Puppa A, et al. Diffusion-weighted imaging does not predict histological grading in meningiomas. Acta Neurochir 2010;152: 1315–9.

24. Sanverdi SE, Ozgen B, Oguz KK, et al. Is diffusion-weighted imaging useful in grading and differentiating histopathological subtypes of meningiomas? Eur J Radiol 2012;81:2389–95.

25. Kinoshita Y, Kajiwara H, Yokota A, et al. Proton magnetic resonance spectroscopy of brain tumors: an in vitro study. Neurosurgery 1994;35(4):606–14.

26. Demir MK, Iplikcioglu AC, Dincer A, et al. Single voxel proton MR spectroscopy findings of typical and atypical intracranial meningiomas. Eur J Radiol 2006;60:48–55.

27. Kousi E, Tsougos I, Fountas K, et al. Distinct peak at 3.8 ppm observed by 3T MR spectroscopy in meningiomas, while nearly absent in high-grade gliomas and cerebral metastasis. Mol Med Rep 2012;5: 1011–8.

28. Pfisterer WK, Hendricks WP, Scheck AC, et al. Fluorescent in situ hybridization and ex vivo 1H magnetic resonance spectroscopic examinations of meningioma tumor tissue: is it possible to identify a clinically-aggressive subset of benign meningiomas? Neurosurgery 2007;61(5):1048–61.

29. Tugnoli V, Schenetti L, Mucci A, et al. Ex vivo HR-MAS MRS of human meningiomas: a comparison with in vivo 1H MR spectra. Int J Mol Med 2006;18: 859–69.

30. Kanberoglu B, Moore NZ, Frakes D, et al. Neuronavigation using three-dimensional proton magnetic resonance spectroscopy data. Stereotact Funct Neurosurg 2014;92:306–14.

31. Valotassiou V, Leondi A, Angelidis G, et al. SPECT and PET imaging of meningiomas. ScientificWorldJournal 2012;2012:412580.

32. Afshar-Oromieh A, Wolf MB, Kratochwil C, et al. Comparison of 68Ga-DOTATOC-PET/CT and PET/MR hybrid systems in patients with cranial meningiomas: initial results. Neuro Oncol 2015;17(2):312–9.

Predicting Meningioma Consistency on Preoperative Neuroimaging Studies

Mark S. Shiroishi, MD[a,*], Steven Y. Cen, PhD[a],
Benita Tamrazi, MD[b], Francesco D'Amore, MD[a],
Alexander Lerner, MD[a], Kevin S. King, MD[a],
Paul E. Kim, MD[a], Meng Law, MD[a], Darryl H. Hwang, PhD[a],
Orest B. Boyko, MD, PhD[a], Chia-Shang J. Liu, MD, PhD[a]

KEYWORDS

- Meningioma • Consistency • Firmness • Texture • MRI • Prediction • Neurosurgical planning
- Minimally invasive neurosurgery

KEY POINTS

- There are currently no validated neuroimaging techniques to predict preoperative meningioma consistency.
- T2-weighted imaging evaluation is relatively straightforward and may be useful. However, further validation is needed.
- Little is known about advanced MRI techniques, such as diffusion MRI, magnetic resonance (MR) elastography (MRE), and MR spectroscopy. Of these techniques, MRE and diffusion tensor imaging appear particularly promising.

INTRODUCTION

Meningioma is the most common primary brain tumor.[1] With surgery being a primary mode of therapy, minimally invasive alternatives to conventional open approaches to the resection of intracranial meningiomas, such as keyhole or endoscopic transnasal approaches, have recently become more commonplace in tumors of the skull base.[2–5] However, proper patient selection is critical to determine which neurosurgical operation is most appropriate for a given patient. Multiple factors, such as tumor location, invasiveness, encasement of vital structures, and vascularity, must be taken into consideration.[3,6–8] Tumor consistency, also referred to as firmness or texture, is another factor that has been increasingly recognized as an important criterion to consider before a meningioma operation. Multiple reports have described the significance of a meningioma's consistency to determine surgical planning and expectations regarding the extent of resection.[3,9–13] Furthermore, this information can be very helpful when patients are counseled regarding potential risks and length of operating time.[14] This is particularly true for tumors that demonstrate extremes of consistency (ie, extremely soft vs extremely firm). Although it appears that water and collagen content are important determinants

Funding: M.S. Shiroishi is supported in part by SC CTSI (NIH/NCRR/NCATS) Grant KL2TR000131, Toshiba American Medical Systems; he is also a consultant for Guerbet.
[a] Department of Radiology, Keck School of Medicine, University of Southern California, Los Angeles, CA 90033, USA; [b] Pediatric Neuroradiology, Children's Hospital Los Angeles, Keck School of Medicine, University of Southern California, Los Angeles, CA 90027, USA
* Corresponding author.
E-mail address: Mark.Shiroishi@med.usc.edu

neurosurgery.theclinics.com

of meningioma consistency, no definite association with histopathological subtype has been established.[2,5–7,15–17] This review summarizes the current neuroimaging literature as it relates to the preoperative evaluation of meningioma consistency.

REFERENCE STANDARDS OF MENINGIOMA CONSISTENCY

Before delving into the neuroimaging aspects of meningioma consistency determination, it is necessary to consider what reference standards are being used when a neuroimaging method is being evaluated for its discriminative ability. In 2013, Zada and colleagues[2] proposed a meningioma consistency grading system based on an ordinal scale rather than simply labeling meningiomas as either "soft" or "hard." The impetus for their approach was due to the common practice in neuroimaging studies of *retrospectively* using this binary approach based on neurosurgical operative reports, a method that also failed to recognize areas of mixed consistency within the tumor. Their 5-point scale was based on the surgeon's ability to internally debulk the meningioma as well as the ease with which the tumor capsule could be folded after debulking. A grade of 1 corresponded to an extremely soft tumor that required only suction for internal debulking and either had no capsule or the capsule was easily folded. At the other extreme, a 5 represented a calcified, extremely firm tumor with a density that was close to that of bone and whose rigid capsule did not allow for collapse or folding. Debulking of these tumors was difficult despite the use of ultrasonic aspiration, cautery loop, or sharp/mechanical dissection. Using this scale, 2 neurosurgeons independently evaluated 50 consecutive patients with meningioma who underwent surgical resection in a *prospective* fashion. The investigators found that this proposed grading system resulted in a high degree of user agreement between the 2 surgeons for overall tumor consistency. The investigators of a very recent neuroimaging study of meningioma consistency felt that the Zada classification resulted in less variability and subjectivity compared with a neurosurgeon's qualitative assessment of "hard" versus "soft."[5] Utilization of grading schemes such as those proposed by Zada and colleagues[2] may allow for more objective comparison of studies examining meningioma consistency.

NEUROIMAGING STUDIES OF MENINGIOMA CONSISTENCY

There have been a variety of neuroimaging approaches that have sought to predict meningioma consistency. However, there have been conflicting results and *no* universally accepted method has been established to date. These studies have used imaging approaches ranging from conventional imaging (MRI, computed tomography [CT]) to the application of advanced MRI techniques (**Box 1**).

Conventional MRI

Most of the literature concerned with imaging prediction of meningioma consistency has used conventional MRI techniques. **Table 1** provides on overview of these studies. To the best of our knowledge, the earliest of these was that by Chen and colleagues[16] from our institution. Their retrospective study of 54 patients found that hyperintensity on T2-weighted imaging (T2WI) relative to gray matter was associated with soft tumor consistency. On the other hand, T1-weighted imaging (T1WI) had no association with consistency. Indeed, multiple other studies have shown that there is an association between signal intensity on T2WI and meningioma consistency.[4,6–9,14,17–21] The hyperintensity on T2WI of soft tumors may be related to higher water content, whereas the lower signal on T2WI for hard tumors might be due to less water and more collagen and calcium content.[5,6,8,16,17,20,21] Increased cellularity is also thought to play a role in decreasing signal intensity on T2WI. Its interaction with fibrous content and interstitial fluid, which may increase signal intensity on T2WI, can affect signal intensity in a complex manner that could limit diagnostic accuracy of meningioma consistency prediction.[22]

Most conventional MRI studies have not found that there is an association between T1WI and meningioma consistency.[4,6–8,16] However, in one study, Hoover and colleagues[14] found that meningiomas that were hyperintense on T2WI and hypointense on T1WI were more likely soft, whereas

---

Box 1
Various neuroimaging techniques that have been examined to predict meningioma consistency

Conventional MRI: mainly T2-weighted imaging

Diffusion MRI: diffusion-weighted imaging and diffusion tensor imaging

Magnetic resonance (MR) spectroscopy

MR elastography

Dynamic contrast-enhanced MRI

Magnetization transfer MRI

Conventional computed tomography

those that were hypointense on T2WI and isointense on T1WI were more likely firm. However, they reported low sensitivity to detect firm tumors. In another study, Ortega-Porcayo and colleagues.[5] found that by using combined T1WI and T2WI signal intensities relative to cerebral cortex were associated very soft or very hard tumors; however, this technique also suffered from low sensitivity for detecting hard tumors.

It is important to note, however, that not all studies have found an association between conventional MRI and meningioma consistency. Carpeggiani and colleagues[23] examined 43 meningiomas and found no correlation between MRI signal intensity and consistency. However, the investigators did feel that soft tumors tended to show hyperintensity on T2WI. Similarly, Kashimura and colleagues[24] found that there was no association between T2WI and consistency. A more recent larger series from Romani and colleagues[25] also found no association using T1WI or T2WI, as well as fluid-attenuated inversion recovery (FLAIR) or proton density–weighted imaging (PDWI). However, several other studies found MRI techniques other than T2WI, like FLAIR and PDWI, were indeed associated with consistency.[4,7,8]

The obvious appeal of using conventional MRI lies in its practicality, as imaging techniques like T2WI are routinely incorporated in standard brain MRI protocols. In its simplest form, signal intensity can be evaluated visually without the need for specialized postprocessing techniques or expertise. **Figs. 1** and **2** demonstrate meningiomas that would be unambiguously categorized as hypointense, isointense, and hyperintense on T2WI; however, it must be kept in mind that evaluation in this way is not quantitative. Reconstructed MRI intensity is based on arbitrary units and direct comparison between different acquisitions cannot be performed. Often, enhanced tissue separation via pulse sequence or hardware design is not only vendor propriety information, but also a competitive marketing advantage for the MR manufacturer. Also, because of its subjective nature, visual evaluation of signal intensity can become difficult (**Fig. 3**). This is particularly true when heterogeneous signal intensities can appear in larger tumors[6,23] (**Fig. 4**). A few studies have incorporated the use of signal intensity ratios comparing the signal intensity of the meningioma relative to the cerebral cortex so as to provide a bit more objectivity to signal intensity assessment.[4,19,21] Also, most of the studies that have found an association between consistency and conventional MRI have not reported measures of diagnostic accuracy; the results of those few that did, do not appear sufficient to support its use in routine clinical practice.[4,5,14,20]

Other factors that could be determined from conventional MRI images, such as contrast enhancement on T1WI, presence of cystic components, peritumoral vasogenic edema, brain-tumor contact interface, or bony appearance, also have not been associated with tumor consistency in several studies.[8,14,20,25] Furthermore, neither angiographic characteristics nor clinical factors, such as gender or age, have been associated with consistency.

Diffusion MRI

Diffusion-weighted imaging (DWI) is a routinely applied functional MRI technique that depends on the microscopic mobility of water to determine tissue contrast. The apparent diffusion coefficient (ADC) provides a measure of water motion in which lower ADC values will be seen in areas of restricted diffusion.[26,28] DWI has found application in a variety of neurologic processes, particularly for the evaluation of cerebral ischemia as well as neoplasms. Although a detailed understanding of the biophysical basis of DWI on a microscopic scale remains incomplete, it is thought that DWI can provide information regarding tissue architecture at the millimeter scale by characterizing impedance of water diffusion due to cellular packing, macromolecules, membranes, and intracellular elements.[26] DWI measures water diffusion as an average of all directions, whereas diffusion tensor imaging (DTI) is a more sophisticated 3-dimensional (3D) Gaussian model–based method that can fit both magnitude and directionality of diffusion to provide insight into the 3D microstructure of the brain parenchyma.[26]

Although DWI is routinely performed during clinical MRI examinations, there has been relatively little work using this to predict meningioma consistency. Presently, the handful of studies that have been performed have produced contradictory results. Hoover and colleagues[14] found that a meningioma's appearance on DWI or its ADC had no association with tumor consistency, whereas T1/T2WI did demonstrate an association. Similar findings were also seen more recently by Watanabe and colleagues,[4] where ADC showed no association and quantitative assessment of T2WI and FLAIR was helpful. On the other hand, Yogi and colleagues[22] found that hard meningiomas contained significantly lower minimum ADC values compared with soft tumors. Using a minimum ADC cutoff value of 0.64×10^{-3} mm^2/s, they reported a sensitivity of 88% and specificity of 81%, and receiver operating characteristic analysis revealed an area under the curve (AUC) of 0.9.

Table 1
Conventional MRI studies that have sought to predict meningioma consistency

Author, Year	No. of Cases	Association Between Conventional MRI and Consistency?	Method of MRI Signal Intensity Determination	Reference Standard for Consistency
Chen et al,[16] 1992	54	Yes, T2WI	Visual	Operative report, described as "soft" or "firm"
Carpeggiani et al,[23] 1993	43	No	Visual	Operative and pathologic report, described as "soft," "hard," or "mixed"
Suzuki et al,[6] 1994	73	Yes, T2WI	Visual	Operative report and video recordings taking into consideration surgical instruments, described as "soft," "moderate," or "hard"
Yamaguchi et al,[7] 1997	50	Yes, T2WI and PDWI	Visual	Intraoperative based on surgical instruments used, described as "soft," "mixed," or "hard"
Maiuri et al,[17] 1997	35	Yes, T2WI	Visual	Pathologic report examining histologic subtype
Yrjänä et al,[19] 2006	21	Yes, T2WI	Relative signal intensities were created by dividing tumor signal intensity by cortical gray matter	Intraoperative based on visual analog scale
Kashimura et al,[24] 2007	29	No	Visual	Intraoperative based on surgical instruments used, described as "soft" or "hard"
Kim et al,[9] 2008	27	Yes, T2WI	Visual	Intraoperative findings, described as "friable soft" or "hard"
Hoover et al,[14] 2011	101	Yes, T1WI and T2WI	Visual	Operative report, described as "soft and/or suckable" or "firm and/or fibrous"

Study	N	Preoperative MRI	Method	Intraoperative assessment
Chernov et al,[20] 2011	49	Yes, T2WI	Visual	Intraoperative based on instruments used, described as "soft," "mixed," or "hard"
Sitthinamsuwan et al,[8] 2012	243	Yes, T2WI and FLAIR	Visual	Intraoperative based on instruments used and video recordings, described as "soft," "intermediate," or "hard"
Romani et al,[25] 2014	110	No	Visual	Intraoperative assessment based on surgical instruments used and tactile sense, described as "soft," "medium," or "hard"
Ortega-Porcayo et al,[5] 2015	16	Yes, T1WI and T2WI	Visual	Intraoperative assessment using Zada et al[2] grading system and dichotomous "soft" or "hard" grading
Smith et al,[21] 2015	20	Yes, T2WI	Used T2WI to create tumor to middle cerebellar peduncle ratios	Intraoperative assessment based on Cavitron Ultrasonic Surgical Aspirator intensity to designate tumors as "soft," "intermediate," or "firm"
Watanabe et al,[4] 2015	43	Yes, T2WI, FLAIR, contrast-enhanced FIESTA	Created signal intensity ratio by comparing tumor to cerebral cortex	Intraoperative based on visual analog scale

Abbreviations: FIESTA, fast imaging employing steady-state acquisition; FLAIR, fluid attenuation inversion recovery imaging; PDWI, proton density–weighted imaging; T1WI, T1-weighted imaging; T2WI, T2-weighted imaging.
Data from Refs.[4–9,14,16,17,19–21,23–25]

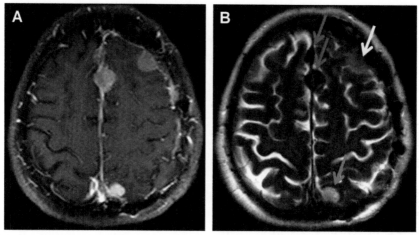

Fig. 1. Multiple meningiomas showing the spectrum of signal intensities on T2WI. Axial contrast-enhanced T1WI (*A*) demonstrates multiple small contrast-enhancing meningiomas. The corresponding axial T2WI (*B*) demonstrates that the 2 meningiomas along the anterior falx show hypointensity relative to gray matter (*red arrows*). The meningioma along the left frontal convexity appears isointense on T2WI (*yellow arrow*) and a small left parietal convexity parafalcine meningioma adjacent to the superior sagittal sinus appears hyperintense on T2WI (*blue arrow*).

The investigators theorized that these results were presumably related to higher cellularity and fibrous content in harder lesions, although they lacked histopathological validation. However, overlap of ADC values was still present, which could limit its use as a determinant of consistency.

In 2007, using the assumption that fibroblastic meningiomas are typically hard in consistency, Tropine and colleagues[15] examined 30 meningiomas using DTI to attempt to distinguish fibroblastic histologic subtypes from other subtypes of meningioma. Fractional anisotropy (FA), as well as geometric shape of the diffusion tensors appeared to be able to differentiate fibroblastic meningiomas from the other types. However, these results were not compared with an actual assessment of meningioma consistency. The same year, Kashimura and colleagues[24] showed that FA values for hard meningiomas were significantly higher compared to soft ones. Using an FA cut-off value of 0.3, they demonstrated sensitivity of 91% and specificity of 67%. Fibrous content has been thought to underlie a given FA value where parallel-oriented cellular membranes result

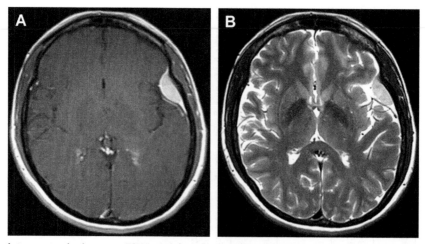

Fig. 2. Hyperintense meningioma on T2WI. Axial contrast-enhanced T1WI (*A*) demonstrates a homogeneously enhancing left fronto-temporal convexity meningioma. Axial T2WI (*B*) shows that the mass appears hyperintense compared to cortex.

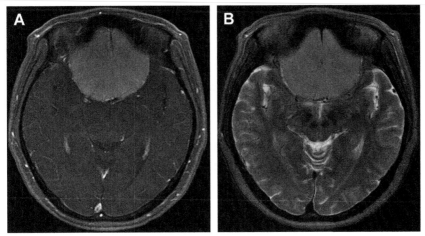

Fig. 3. Isointense to slightly hyperintense meningioma on T2WI. Axial contrast-enhanced T1WI (*A*) demonstrates a large homogeneously enhancing anterior skull-base meningioma. Axial T2WI (*B*) shows this mass appears iso-intense to slightly hyperintense compared with the cortex. The use of subjective visual criteria to classify signal intensity can be problematic in cases such as this.

in diffusion preferentially in one direction while being restricted along other axes.[4] A recent large prospective series of 110 meningiomas by Romani and colleagues[25] also found that the quantitative FA value, as well as signal intensity on FA and mean diffusivity (MD) maps, were predictive of meningioma consistency. Using rigorous statistical methodology with a relatively large sample size, they determined an impressive AUC of 0.9459. Interestingly, these investigators also found that conventional MRI sequences, such as T1WI, T2WI, FLAIR, PDWI, and arterial spin labeling (ASL) perfusion, had no association with consistency (see previously, under Conventional MRI).

However, not all studies are in agreement regarding DTI; Ortega-Porcayo and colleagues[5] found that FA values showed no association with consistency.

Magnetic Resonance Elastography

Magnetic resonance elastography (MRE) is an emerging advanced MRI technique that has promise to determine meningioma consistency. Meant to provide a measure of tissue stiffness akin to manual palpation, MRE has been investigated in other parts of the body.[28] One such application is in the evaluation of hepatic fibrosis, in which

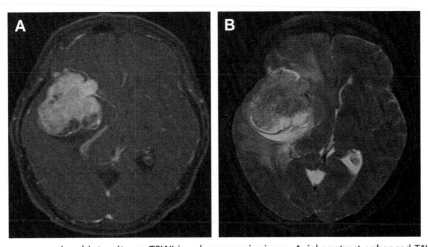

Fig. 4. Heterogeneous signal intensity on T2WI in a large meningioma. Axial contrast-enhanced T1WI (*A*) demonstrates a large heterogeneously enhancing right sphenoid-wing meningioma growing superiorly into the temporoinsular region along with mass effect and midline shift. Axial T2WI (*B*) demonstrates surrounding vasogenic edema and very heterogeneous signal intensity within the mass. Subjective categorization of signal intensity in the face of marked heterogeneity can be difficult.

its use has taken the place of needle biopsies in some centers.[30] In MRE, stiffness is determined by evaluation of shear wave movement through tissue. This is accomplished by applying an external mechanical shear wave and measuring the viscoelastic properties of the tissue.[31] Although the use of MRE in the brain is made technically challenging by several factors, such as the presence of the skull, a few recent publications have examined its utility in determining meningioma consistency.

In 2007, Xu and colleagues[32] used MRE in a series of 6 patients: 4 patients with meningioma and 1 patient each with schwannoma and hemangiopericytoma. Based on intraoperative assessment, 1 meningioma, as well as the schwannoma and hemangiopericytoma, had hard intraoperative consistency, whereas 2 meningiomas had intermediate consistency and 1 meningioma had soft consistency. In this pilot study, their qualitative MRE measurements appeared to agree with intraoperative assessment of consistency. In 2013, Murphy and colleagues[31] performed a prospective study of 13 meningiomas using quantitative MRE stiffness measurements in which MRE measurements were significantly correlated with intraoperative qualitative assessment of tumor consistency. The investigators put forth that a major advantage of MRE is its ability to capture the full spectrum of meningioma consistency (ie, intermediate hardness). On the other hand, conventional measurements based on T1WI and T2WI may best predict only very soft or hard tumors. A subsequent prospective study by the same group used higher-resolution MRE in an attempt to better capture the intratumoral heterogeneity of consistency.[33] They found that higher resolution (3-mm isotropic resolution as opposed to 4 mm performed in Murphy and colleagues[31]), had high specificity and positive predictive value to detect heterogeneity and hard consistency. However, it had low specificity and positive predictive value to rule in homogeneity and soft consistency as well as low sensitivity to rule out hard tumors.

Magnetic Resonance Spectroscopy

Magnetic resonance spectroscopy (MRS) is another advanced MRI functional technique that has been used clinically and in research settings for several decades for many applications, particularly brain tumors.[34,35] Proton (^{1}H)-MRS is the most commonly used MRS technique, and it can provide metabolic data of brain lesions by measuring metabolites such as choline and N-acetyl aspartate, which are involved in membrane synthesis/degradation and neuronal integrity, respectively. Although MRS is not a new technique, there has been very little in the literature regarding its utility to predict meningioma consistency. In 2011, Chernov and colleagues[20] evaluated 100 meningiomas using ^{1}H-MRS, 49 of which had intraoperative consistency data. In this study, no metabolic information from ^{1}H-MRS had an association with meningioma consistency, whereas T2WI did show an association (see **Table 1**).

Computed Tomography

CT scans are ubiquitous in clinical practice and are frequently used in the work-up of patients who may have an intracranial mass. As with diffusion MRI and MRS, very little has been published regarding the use of CT imaging for determining meningioma consistency. In 1979, Kendall and Pullicino[36] reported on a series of 77 meningiomas using both visual and quantitative CT assessment of hard versus soft meningiomas. There was a significant overlap of the CT features between hard versus soft tumors, making differentiation of tumor consistency difficult.[15,31] The more recent study by Hoover and colleagues[14] referred to previously also found that CT showed no association with tumor consistency. Likewise, Sitthinamsuwan and colleagues[8] found that neither contrast-enhanced CT nor calcified composition on noncontrast enhanced CT was associated with consistency.

Other Imaging Techniques

In addition to the imaging methods mentioned previously, a couple of publications have used other advanced MRI techniques in the context of meningioma consistency prediction. The work by Yrjänä and colleagues,[19] mentioned previously in the Conventional MRI section, was one of multiple studies that demonstrated an association of T2WI with meningioma consistency. Their study, which was performed using a low-field 0.23T MRI scanner, also used T1-weighted dynamic contrast-enhanced (DCE) MRI. This technique uses rapid T1WI before, during, and after gadolinium-based contrast agent administration to characterize features associated with microvascular perfusion and permeability of brain lesions such as tumors. The investigators found that no DCE-MRI parameters were correlated with meningioma consistency; however, semiquantitative parameters such as time to maximum enhancement was associated with microvessel density.

Work by Yoneoka and colleagues[37] used a variation of conventional MRI called T2 reversed (T2R) imaging, which takes advantage of high-field MRI with its high signal-to-noise ratio with gray-scale reversal to improve contrast resolution.[38] Using T2R imaging, they showed that differences in T2R heterogeneity were associated with meningioma consistency.

Magnetization transfer (MT) imaging is an advanced MRI technique that can generate unique contrast in tissues not obtainable with standard techniques. MT imaging depends on the use of off-resonance radiofrequency pulses in which a magnetization transfer ratio (MTR) can be determined by measuring signal intensity with and without the off-resonance pulse.[39,40] In 1999, Okumura applied MT imaging in meningiomas and a variety of other brain tumors and found that there was a significant difference in MTR between soft and hard tumors.[41]

SUMMARY

This review has summarized the neuroimaging literature focused on preoperative prediction of meningioma consistency. A diagnostically accurate and robust technique would provide critical information that can guide the neurosurgical decision-making and inform patients and their families regarding risks and expectations. Thus far, most work has focused on conventional MRI methods, and although there have been multiple articles showing the promise of T2WI to predict consistency, it is still not a validated method. Most studies have small sample sizes, many are retrospective, and not all studies are in agreement. The actual diagnostic accuracy is not known in most studies, and in those cases in which it has been reported, there is often poor sensitivity and/or specificity.[31] In addition, other factors, such as variations in MRI scanners and acquisition parameters and methodological issues relating to qualitative versus quantitative analysis, variations in reference standards of consistency and other differences in data analysis can potentially limit the internal as well as the external validity of these studies. Future, well-powered, prospective multicenter imaging studies are needed to validate these and other neuroimaging methods. Similar issues are also concerns for more advanced MRI techniques, such as diffusion MRI, MRE, and MRS, in which there is a relative paucity of data compared with conventional MRI methods. Of these methods, MRE and DTI appear particularly promising and deserve further rigorous examination.

REFERENCES

1. Rogers L, Barani I, Chamberlain M, et al. Meningiomas: knowledge base, treatment outcomes, and uncertainties. A RANO review. J Neurosurg 2015; 122(1):4–23.
2. Zada G, Yashar P, Robison A, et al. A proposed grading system for standardizing tumor consistency of intracranial meningiomas. Neurosurg Focus 2013; 35(6):E1.
3. Zada G, Du R, Laws ER Jr. Defining the "edge of the envelope": patient selection in treating complex sellar-based neoplasms via transsphenoidal versus open craniotomy. J Neurosurg 2011;114(2): 286–300.
4. Watanabe K, Kakeda S, Yamamoto J, et al. Prediction of hard meningiomas: quantitative evaluation based on the magnetic resonance signal intensity. Acta Radiol 2015. [Epub ahead of print].
5. Ortega-Porcayo LA, Ballesteros-Zebadua P, Marrufo-Melendez OR, et al. Prediction of mechanical properties and subjective consistency of meningiomas using T1-T2 assessment vs Fractional Anisotropy. World Neurosurg 2015. [Epub ahead of print].
6. Suzuki Y, Sugimoto T, Shibuya M, et al. Meningiomas: correlation between MRI characteristics and operative findings including consistency. Acta Neurochir (Wien) 1994;129(1–2):39–46.
7. Yamaguchi N, Kawase T, Sagoh M, et al. Prediction of consistency of meningiomas with preoperative magnetic resonance imaging. Surg Neurol 1997; 48(6):579–83.
8. Sitthinamsuwan B, Khampalikit I, Nunta-aree S, et al. Predictors of meningioma consistency: a study in 243 consecutive cases. Acta Neurochir (Wien) 2012;154(8):1383–9.
9. Kim TW, Jung S, Jung TY, et al. Prognostic factors of postoperative visual outcomes in tuberculum sellae meningioma. Br J Neurosurg 2008;22:231–4.
10. Little KM, Friedman AH, Sampson JH, et al. Surgical management of petroclival meningiomas: defining resection goals based on risk of neurological morbidity and tumor recurrence rates in 137 patients. Neurosurgery 2005;56(3):546–59 [discussion: 546–59].
11. Sekhar LN, Jannetta PJ, Burkhart LE, et al. Meningiomas involving the clivus: a six-year experience with 41 patients. Neurosurgery 1990;27(5):764–81 [discussion: 781].
12. Tahara A, de Santana PA Jr, Calfat Maldaun MV, et al. Petroclival meningiomas: surgical management and common complications. J Clin Neurosci 2009;16(5):655–9.
13. Fahlbusch R, Schott W. Pterional surgery of meningiomas of the tuberculum sellae and planum sphenoidale: surgical results with special consideration of ophthalmological and endocrinological outcomes. J Neurosurg 2002;96(2):235–43.
14. Kelly PJ. "Magnetic resonance imaging and meningiomas". Commentary to Hoover JM, Morris JM,

Meyer FB. Use of preoperative magnetic resonance imaging T1 and T2 sequences to determine intraoperative meningioma consistency. Surg Neurol Int 2011;2:142.

15. Tropine A, Dellani PD, Glaser M, et al. Differentiation of fibroblastic meningiomas from other benign subtypes using diffusion tensor imaging. J Magn Reson Imaging 2007;25(4):703–8.

16. Chen TC, Zee CS, Miller CA, et al. Magnetic resonance imaging and pathological correlates of meningiomas. Neurosurgery 1992;31(6):1015–21 [discussion: 1021–2].

17. Maiuri F, Iaconetta G, de Divitiis O, et al. Intracranial meningiomas: correlations between MR imaging and histology. Eur J Radiol 1999;31(1):69–75.

18. Zee CS, Chin T, Segall HD, et al. Magnetic resonance imaging of meningiomas. Semin Ultrasound CT MR 1992;13(3):154–69.

19. Yrjänä SK, Tuominen H, Karttunen A, et al. Low-field MR imaging of meningiomas including dynamic contrast enhancement study: evaluation of surgical and histopathologic characteristics. AJNR Am J Neuroradiol 2006;27(10):2128–34.

20. Chernov MF, Kasuya H, Nakaya K, et al. ^{1}H-MRS of intracranial meningiomas: what it can add to known clinical and MRI predictors of the histopathological and biological characteristics of the tumor? Clin Neurol Neurosurg 2011;113(3):202–12.

21. Smith KA, Leever JD, Chamoun RB. Predicting consistency of meningioma by magnetic resonance imaging. J Neurol Surg B Skull Base 2015;76(3):225–9.

22. Yogi A, Koga T, Azama K, et al. Usefulness of the apparent diffusion coefficient (ADC) for predicting the consistency of intracranial meningiomas. Clin Imaging 2014;38(6):802–7.

23. Carpeggiani P, Crisi G, Trevisan C. MRI of intracranial meningiomas: correlations with histology and physical consistency. Neuroradiology 1993;35(7):532–6.

24. Kashimura H, Inoue T, Ogasawara K, et al. Prediction of meningioma consistency using fractional anisotropy value measured by magnetic resonance imaging. J Neurosurg 2007;107(4):784–7.

25. Romani R, Tang WJ, Mao Y, et al. Diffusion tensor magnetic resonance imaging for predicting the consistency of intracranial meningiomas. Acta Neurochir (Wien) 2014;156(10):1837–45.

26. Padhani AR, Liu G, Koh DM, et al. Diffusion-weighted magnetic resonance imaging as a cancer biomarker: consensus and recommendations. Neoplasia 2009;11(2):102–25.

27. Shiroishi MS, Boxerman JL, Pope WB. Physiologic MRI for assessment of response to therapy and prognosis in glioblastoma. Neuro Oncol 2015. [Epub ahead of print].

28. Lerner A, Mogensen MA, Kim PE, et al. Clinical applications of diffusion tensor imaging. World Neurosurg 2014;82(1–2):96–109.

29. Muthupillai R, Lomas DJ, Rossman PJ, et al. Magnetic resonance elastography by direct visualization of propagating acoustic strain waves. Science 1995;269(5232):1854–7.

30. Yin M, Woollard J, Wang X, et al. Quantitative assessment of hepatic fibrosis in an animal model with magnetic resonance elastography. Magn Reson Med 2007;58(2):346–53.

31. Murphy MC, Huston J 3rd, Glaser KJ, et al. Preoperative assessment of meningioma stiffness using magnetic resonance elastography. J Neurosurg 2013;118(3):643–8.

32. Xu L, Lin Y, Han JC, et al. Magnetic resonance elastography of brain tumors: preliminary results. Acta Radiol 2007;48(3):327–30.

33. Hughes JD, Fattahi N, Van Gompel J, et al. Higher-resolution magnetic resonance elastography in meningiomas to determine intratumoral consistency. Neurosurgery 2015;77(4):653–9.

34. Bottomley PA, Edelstein WA, Foster TH, et al. In vivo solvent-suppressed localized hydrogen nuclear magnetic resonance spectroscopy: a window to metabolism? Proc Natl Acad Sci U S A 1985;82(7):2148–52.

35. Horska A, Barker PB. Imaging of brain tumors: MR spectroscopy and metabolic imaging. Neuroimaging Clin N Am 2010;20(3):293–310.

36. Kendall B, Pullicino P. Comparison of consistency of meningiomas and CT appearances. Neuroradiology 1979;18(4):173–6.

37. Yoneoka Y, Fujii Y, Takahashi H, et al. Pre-operative histopathological evaluation of meningiomas by 3 0T T2R MRI. Acta Neurochir (Wien) 2002;144(10):953–7 [discussion: 957].

38. Fujii Y, Nakayama N, Nakada T. High-resolution T2-reversed magnetic resonance imaging on a high magnetic field system. Technical note. J Neurosurg 1998;89(3):492–5.

39. Henkelman RM, Stanisz GJ, Graham SJ. Magnetization transfer in MRI: a review. NMR Biomed 2001;14(2):57–64.

40. Grossman RI, Gomori JM, Ramer KN, et al. Magnetization transfer: theory and clinical applications in neuroradiology. Radiographics 1994;14(2):279–90.

41. Okumura A, Takenaka K, Nishimura Y, et al. The characterization of human brain tumor using magnetization transfer technique in magnetic resonance imaging. Neurol Res 1999;21(3):250–4.

Strategic and Technical Considerations for the Endovascular Embolization of Intracranial Meningiomas

Robert F. James, MD[a], Daniel R. Kramer, MD[b], Paul S. Page, BS[a], John R. Gaughen Jr, MD[c], Lacey B. Martin, MD[d], William J. Mack, MD[b],*

KEYWORDS

- Meningioma • Endovascular • Embolization • Technique • Dangerous anastomoses

KEY POINTS

- Endovascular embolization can be used as an adjunct to surgical resection of meningiomas.
- Meningiomas that may benefit most from embolization are large, vascular tumors in surgically challenging locations.
- Critical endpoints for assessment of embolization efficacy are difficult to quantify.
- Optimal timing of endovascular embolization remains unclear.

INTRODUCTION: NATURE OF THE PROBLEM

Meningiomas comprise approximately 15% to 20% of all intracranial tumors.[1–3] Although small incidental tumors can be followed,[4,5] larger, symptomatic tumors are most often treated with a goal of curative gross total resection and symptom resolution.[1] However, meningioma resection is not benign. Surgical morbidity has been shown to be 30% and mortality 4% in the general population[6] and 48% and 6.6%, respectively, in the elderly.[7] Preoperative endovascular embolization has been advocated to reduce intraoperative blood loss and improve ease of surgical resection.[1,8] Embolization of tumor arteries, not anatomically accessible during the surgical approach, may be of benefit to the surgeon. Tumor softening and necrosis after embolization may aid in the resection of firm tumors and decrease the need for brain retraction within confined operative corridors. On rare occasions, therapeutic embolization can be performed to prevent tumor growth and/or decrease tumor burden. The role for such palliative embolization should be restricted to poor candidates for surgery with extensive comorbidities.[9,10]

Despite refinement in catheters, wires, and embolic agents, complications still occur during preoperative embolization of meningiomas. Because the procedure is not typically curative, concerns over the usefulness of this treatment

Conflict of Interest: No funding was received for this, and no conflict of interest exists among any of the authors.
[a] Department of Neurosurgery, University of Louisville School of Medicine, 550 S. Jackson St., Louisville, KY 40204, USA; [b] Department of Neurosurgery, University of Southern California Keck School of Medicine, 1520 San Pablo Street, Suite 3800, Los Angeles, CA 90089, USA; [c] Department of Radiology and Medical Imaging, University of Virginia Health System, 1215 Lee St., Charlottesville, VA 22908, USA; [d] Department of Neurosurgery, University of Oklahoma School of Medicine, 660 Parrington Oval, Norman, OK 73019, USA
* Corresponding author. USC Department of Neurosurgery, 1520 San Pablo Street, Suite 3800, Los Angeles, CA 90033.
E-mail address: William.Mack@med.usc.edu

Neurosurg Clin N Am 27 (2016) 155–166
http://dx.doi.org/10.1016/j.nec.2015.11.005

have been raised and warrant further investigation.[11] Here we review the decision-making processes and technical considerations that help guide preoperative embolization of meningiomas.

INDICATIONS AND CONTRAINDICATIONS

Little consensus exists as to which meningiomas benefit most from preoperative embolization. Focusing on intraoperative blood loss, reports have suggested that embolization may be most beneficial in meningiomas greater than 5 cm, those that demonstrate a multidirectional external carotid artery (ECA) blood supply, and tumors that possess substantial vascularity[3,11–14] Tumors in anatomically challenging locations, including the middle cranial fossa, sphenoid wing, and paracavernous region may also benefit. Tumors with dural and/or sinus involvement warrant consideration for preoperative embolization.

Studies suggest that preoperative embolization is highly effective in cases of exclusively ECA supply. However, tumors harboring mixed vascular supply with predominantly external contribution also benefit from embolization. Embolization of the ECA feeders serving tumors with mixed vascular supply may result in increased blood flow from the vessels of the internal carotid artery (ICA). This change in flow pattern may negate, or even reverse, the beneficial effects of embolization on blood loss and surgical complexity.[14] Tumors supplied exclusively by branches of the ICA are not ideal for preoperative embolization owing the difficulty involved in safe catheterization and the presence of en passage vessels.[3,12,14]

OPERATIVE TECHNIQUE AND PROCEDURE
Preoperative Planning

A thorough preoperative medical history, detailed neurologic examination, and appropriate serologic analysis can reveal a contrast allergy or renal insufficiency before catheter angiography. Premedication, hydration, and/or minimization of contrast agent may be warranted in these patient populations. Patients often present to the neurosurgeon with a basic MRI study. However, in some cases (sella region, cerebellopontine angle), a fine cut MRI, with and without contrast, is useful for precise anatomic tumor localization. A computed tomography scan may be beneficial in identifying lesional calcifications. These studies will guide both the operative planning and the determinations of whether or not to evaluate the tumor angiographically. Surgeons can consider preoperative MRI or computed tomography angiography to help elucidate whether the tumor may benefit

from embolization before submitting the patient to the risks of catheter angiography.

A preoperative diagnostic catheter angiogram should include, as appropriate, selective evaluation of the ECA, ICA, vertebral arteries, and, if location of the tumor warrants, the thyrocervical and costocervical trunks (typically cervicomedullary or spinal tumors). A bilateral evaluation is critical for parasagittal tumors, because they can recruit blood supply from both sides (**Fig. 1**). Detailed angiographic information assists in guiding the embolization and aids the surgeon with preoperative planning (eg, identification of arterial feeders to be encountered and patency of dural sinuses). Often, the arterial pedicles directly supplying the meningioma must be selected to identify anastomoses that place cranial nerves and key structures at risk during embolization (discussed elsewhere in this paper).

The blood supply to meningiomas arises from the ECA in addition to dural branches of the vertebral and ICA. However, meningiomas can also recruit substantial supply from cortical, pial, and/or scalp–transosseous arteries (see **Fig. 1**). Typically, meningiomas exhibit an intense vascular tumor blush that lasts through the late venous phase on angiography. Superselective angiography of feeding arteries often demonstrates a "sunburst" pattern of tumor staining.[2]

PROCEDURAL CONSIDERATIONS
Timing

Once it is decided to undertake preoperative meningioma embolization, the next consideration is timing. Although no consensus exists, most authors suggest that preoperative embolization should take place shortly before open resection, typically within a few days. Should embolization be performed on the same day as resection, it is prudent to examine the patient's neurologic function between procedures. One study supports delaying surgical resection for at least 24 hours after embolization, exhibiting a reduction in blood loss after a 24-hour delay; however, optimal latency was not quantified.[8] Kai and colleagues[15] propose that the optimal duration between embolization and resection may be 7 to 9 days. The group demonstrates maximal tumor softening, decreased operative times, and lower Simpson grades at this delayed time point. A similar study compared 16 patients with tumor embolization 7 days or greater from the time of resection with a group of 12 patients who underwent surgery less than 7 days from embolization. The authors showed greater reduction in surgical time and blood transfusion volume in the delayed embolization group.[16] However, delayed resection also may

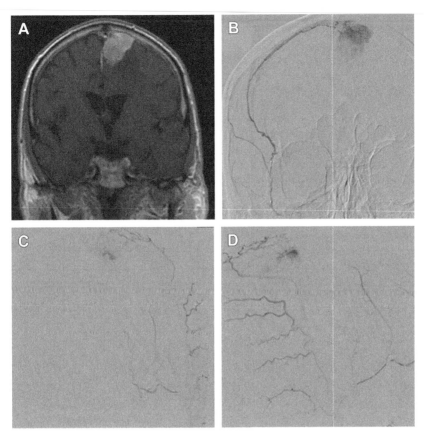

Fig. 1. Parasagittal convexity meningioma. (*A*) Coronal MRI with contrast. (*B*) Superselective angiogram in the anteroposterior (AP) projection of the right middle meningeal artery illustrating contralateral vascular supply that crosses the midline. (*C*) AP and (*D*) lateral superselective angiograms of the left superficial temporal artery demonstrating transosseous vascular supply to the tumor. (*From* Mack WJ, Vinuela F. Diagnostic evaluation and embolization of meningiomas. In: De Monte F, McDermott MW, Al Mefty O, editors. Al- Mefty's meningiomas. 2nd edition. New York: Thieme; 2011. p. 123. Available at: www.thieme.com; with permission.)

allow for tumoral edema and resultant mass effect. Smaller particles (60–150 μm) have better tumor penetration, but can also increase the risk of swelling.[17] This should be considered, especially in the setting of delayed tumor resection. A course of steroids during and after procedures involving high tumor volumes may be warranted; however, the surgeon should still be prepared for emergent decompression and resection if tumoral edema results in neurologic decline, new cranial nerve deficits attributable to compression, or significant mass effect on follow-up imaging.[17,18] Postembolization tumoral edema can be expected anywhere from a few hours to several days after and the patient should be watched closely, particularly in high-risk tumor locations ,such as the posterior or middle fossa.

Preparation and Patient Positioning

The biplane digital subtraction fluoroscopy suite should be prepared in a similar fashion as for any neuroendovascular procedure. Anesthesia options include intravenous sedation, monitored anesthesia care, and general endotracheal anesthesia. When the sedation or monitored anesthesia care option is selected, precise angiographic evaluation of very small dangerous anastomotic channels immediately before embolization requires an extremely cooperative patient who can remain still during image acquisition. If the patient is under general anesthesia, electrophysiologic monitoring can increase procedural safety.

SURGICAL APPROACH AND SURGICAL PROCEDURE
Endovascular Technique

Once ready for embolization, a microcatheter and microguidewire are navigated coaxially through the guide catheter, and distally into the arterial pedicle through which embolization is planned. A microcatheter injection can be performed to identify the microanatomic angioarchitecture of the arterial supply to the meningioma. Microangiography can also aide in the identification of any dangerous anastomoses or blood supply to at-risk cranial nerves. The microcatheter is then navigated more distally, beyond any concerning anatomy, to a position as close as possible to the tumor vascular bed (**Fig. 2**). Reflux of contrast proximally along the catheter is evaluated. Such contrast reflux can predict the potential for reflux of embolic agents. Thus, identification can help to prevent unwanted embolization of more proximally located high-risk branches or the parent artery. Provocative testing with injection of amytal and/or lidocaine can help to identify possible complications of embolization. Either neuromonitoring or immediate neurologic examination helps to identify the effect of the provocative testing.[1]

Next, embolic material is chosen and, with the catheter in good position, it is injected into the tumor. This injection should be done slowly and under biplane fluoroscopy with close monitoring on both planes for reflux or aberrant flow of embolic material. If this occurs, injection should cease immediately. Embolization should continue until the embolic material fails to reach the tumor or unwanted reflux is noted. If particles are used, then embolization continues until slow or stagnant flow is seen in the feeding vessel. Often, embolization can lead to complete, or near complete, angiographic tumor devascularization without selection of all feeding vessels (see **Fig. 2**). If inadequate embolization occurs, further selection of vessels may be necessary. Upon completion of embolization, proximal contrast injection is warranted to assess the entire vascular tree.

SELECTION OF AN EMBOLIC AGENT
Particles

A suspension of particles mixed with contrast agent is most common, offering good penetration and ease of use. Several types of particles of

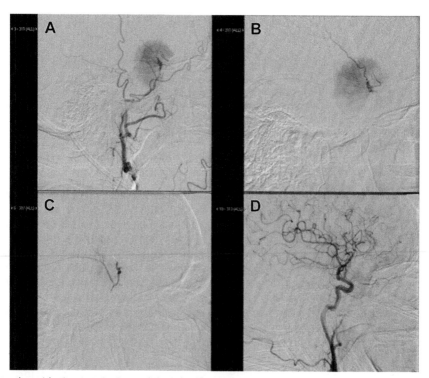

Fig. 2. Right sphenoid wing meningioma. (*A*) Right external carotid artery and (*B*) selective right middle meningeal artery angiograms demonstrate the characteristic vascular blush of a right sphenoid wing meningioma, deriving arterial supply predominantly from branches of the right middle meningeal artery. Note no choroidal blush from these injections. (*C*) Selective right middle meningeal artery angiogram after transarterial embolization of the tumor using polyvinyl alcohol 150 to 250 and 250 to 355 micron particles, resulting in significant devascularization of the meningioma. (*D*) Right common carotid artery angiogram after subsequent coil embolization of the distal right middle meningeal artery trunk demonstrates near-complete devascularization of the tumor and truncation of the right middle meningeal artery. Note a small amount of residual vascular tumor blush arising from branches of the right inferolateral trunk off the cavernous segment of the right internal carotid artery.

varying sizes are available for embolization. The type of particle varies in its visualization, compressibility, subsequent recovery, and ability to aggregate. Each of these factors impacts the choice of agent. Polyvinyl alcohol (PVA) particles are a common choice and available in preparations in a variety of predetermined size ranges. Recognized limitations include difficulty with aggregation, which can lead to microcatheter obstruction. If stoppage occurs, forced injection to clear the catheter is not recommended, because undesired embolization can result. Although smaller PVA particles have shown a greater ability to cause tumor necrosis owing to deeper penetration,[19] smaller size also increases the risk for aberrant embolization to cranial nerves and other critical structures. In a larger observational study, the sole independent risk factor for complications, including cranial nerve deficits and tumor hemorrhage, was small particle size (45–150 μm).[18] Particle size smaller than 150 μm

is thought to increase the risk of embolization to the vasa nervorum of the cranial nerves.[18,20] In most situations, particles with a diameter between 150 and 350 μm will provide optimal tumor penetration and decreased risk for undesired embolization. Tumors with higher flow input may require even larger particles (>500 μm), or an alternative strategy such as gelfoam, liquid embolic agents, or coils (**Fig. 3**).

Made of tris-acryl and cellulose porous beads, microspheres have advantages and disadvantages when compared with PVA particles. The shape and size are more consistent, leaving less variability in advertised size. Additionally, they are more compressible than PVA particles, which helps to prevent the blockage of catheters.[21,22] However, compressibility can also increase the risk of advancement into small vessels serving cranial nerves. One study comparing the 2 types of particles indicated that microspheres exhibited less intraoperative blood loss.[23]

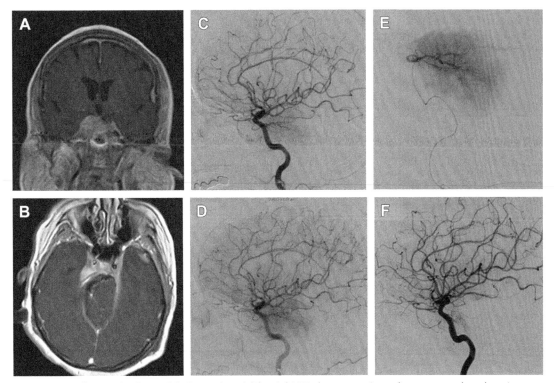

Fig. 3. Suprasellar meningioma. (*A*) Coronal and (*B*) axial MRI demonstrating a homogenously enhancing mass that encases the bilateral internal carotid arteries. Lateral right internal carotid artery angiograms in the (*C*) arterial and (*D*) capillary phases demonstrating a suprasellar tumor blush supplied b enlarged dural branches of the meningohypophyseal trunk. (*E*) Superselective angiogram of the meningohypophyseal trunk. (*F*) A significant decrease in size and intensity of the tumor blush after polyvinyl alcohol and coil embolization of the meningohypophyseal branch supplying the tumor. (*From* Mack WJ, Vinuela F. Diagnostic evaluation and embolization of meningiomas. In: De Monte F, McDermott MW, Al-Mefty O, editors. Al- Mefty's meningiomas. 2nd edition. New York: Thieme; 2011. p. 128. Available at: www.thieme.com; with permission.)

Liquid Embolic Agents

N-Butyl cyanoacrylate (NBCA; TRUFILL, Codman & Shurtleff, Inc, Raynham, MA) and ethylene vinyl alcohol (Onyx; Covidien-ev3 Neurovascular, Irvine, CA) are suspended polymers that solidify when they come into contact with blood. Liquid embolic agents can penetrate into small tumor vessels and are less likely than particles to result in recanalization over time. However, these agents can polymerize within the catheter, can penetrate into small anastomotic vessels, and cost more than particles. The operator must also be cognizant of potential catheter retention with long injections or tortuous anatomy. NBCA is mixed with ethiodol to various dilutions, which allows alteration of the rate of polymerization. Angiographic visibility is increased by adjustment of concentrations or addition of tantalum. Proper embolization with NBCA requires familiarity with the preparation. Advanced technical strategies, such as using coils to obstruct origins to dangerous anastomoses, can help to prevent inadvertent embolization of undesired areas.[24] Advantages of Onyx include an ability to penetrate into tumor capillaries, predictability of solidification, deliberate and controlled injections, and radioopacity.[25] In a small series, of meningiomas, no postembolization tumor edema or hemorrhagic complications were noted.[26]

Other Embolic Agents

Additional agents have been used in meningioma embolization, but reports are limited. These include fibrin glue, ethyl alcohol, hydroxyapatite ceramics, phenytoin, hyperosmolar mannitol, and lipiodol.[27–32] Although virtually all agents show good tumor penetration, each has advantages and disadvantages.

DANGEROUS ANASTOMOSES

Knowledge of potential dangerous extracranial to intracranial anastomoses is critical for safe preoperative tumor embolization, particularly in high-risk areas such as the skull base and orbit (**Table 1**).[2]

Orbital Region

Tumors in the orbital region may have dangerous anastomoses with the central retinal artery branch of the ophthalmic artery (OA). Inadvertent embolization can result in blindness. Less than 1% of the time, the OA arises directly from the meningoophthalmic branch of the middle meningeal artery (MMA), a remnant of the primitive stapedial artery, which increases the risk.[33] A lack of OA visualization on the ICA injection or a choroidal blush identified on superselection of ECA vessels suggests increased risk of vision loss.[34]

Common collaterals to the OA include the anterior and posterior ethmoidal artery branches that anastomose with the ECA circulation via the septal arteries (MMA and sphenopalatine branches of the internal maxillary artery [IMA]). The posterior ethmoidal arteries can also anastomose with the greater palatine artery of the IMA. Additionally, the lacrimal arteries connect with the ECA via the recurrent branch of the MMA through the superior orbital fissure and with the anterior deep temporal and infraorbital arteries of the IMA. The supraorbital artery can arise from the OA and anastomose with the superficial temporal artery. Finally, the dorsal nasal artery, a terminal branch of the OA, connects to the infraorbital artery and the angular branch of the facial artery.[33,34]

Parasellar Region

Meningiomas of the parasellar, sellar, cavernous, or sphenoid wing region often anastomose with the ECA to the cavernous portion of the ICA placing cavernous sinus cranial nerves and ICA supplied cortex at risk.[2] The cavernous portion of the ICA has 3 principal named branches/trunks: the McConnell capsular arteries, the meningohypophyseal trunk, and the inferolateral trunk (ILT). The ILT (also known as the artery of the inferior cavernous sinus) is the most relevant branch to consider for dangerous anastomoses in the setting of parasellar meningiomas (see **Fig. 3**).[34–36] Dangerous anastomoses associated with the ILT invariably arise from branches of the IMA that supply portions of the nearby dural based parasellar meningiomas. These dangerous branches include the superior division of the accessory meningeal artery to the posteromedial branch of the ILT via the foramen ovale, branches of the proximal IMA along the roof of the cavernous sinus to the superior or tentorial branches of the ILT, the artery of the foramen rotundum from the IMA to the anteromedial branch of the ILT, and branches of the OA that traverse the superior orbital fissure to the anteromedial branch of the ILT.[34,36]

Petroclival Region

Meningiomas of the petrous region can develop an ECA supply with anastomotic branches to the ICA via the mandibular artery and the caroticotympanic artery. Likewise, meningiomas of the clival region can have an ECA supply that anastomoses with the ICA through the lateral clival artery and the meningohypophyseal trunk.[34,36]

The pharyngeal and neuromeningeal trunks of the ascending pharyngeal artery are particularly

Table 1
Summary of extracranial and intracranial anastomoses

Extracranial		Intracranial	
Parent Vessel	Major Branch	Minor Branch(es)	Parent Vessel
Internal maxillary	MMA	Orbital branches, anterior branch (anterior falcine)	Ophthalmic
	—	Cavernous branches (posterolateral collateral), temporal rami (anterolateral collateral)	ILT
	—	Petrous branch	CN VII supply
	AMA	Artery of foramen ovale	ILT
	Vidian	—	Petrous ICA
	Artery of foramen rotundum	Anterolateral collateral	ILT
	Anterior deep temporal artery	—	Ophthalmic
Superficial temporal	—	Supraorbital branch	Ophthalmic
Ascending pharyngeal	Superior pharyngeal	Carotid branch (foramen lacerum)	Lateral clival to meningohypophyseal trunk
	—	—	ILT
	Inferior tympanic	—	Caroticotympanic
	Odontoid arch	—	Vertebral artery (C1)
	Hypoglossal and jugular branch	—	Meningohypophyseal trunk of ICA
Posterior auricular–occipital	—	—	CN VII supply
Occipital	—	—	Vertebral artery (C1-C2)
Ascending and deep cervical arteries	—	—	Vertebral artery (C3-C7)

Abbreviations: AMA, accessory meningeal artery; CN, cranial nerve; ICA, internal carotid artery; ILT, inferior lateral trunk; MMA, middle meningeal artery.
   Data from Refs.[27,35,37]

hazardous. Anteriorly, the superior pharyngeal artery, off the pharyngeal trunk, connects to the anastomotic circle of the Eustachian tube. This connects the accessory meningeal artery and pterygovaginal artery (distal branch of IMA) to the petrous ICA mandibular branch. A branch also traverses the foramen lacerum to the carotid canal then enters the cavernous sinus to anastomose with the ICA via the ILT, as well as the recurrent artery of the foramen lacerum. The hypoglossal and jugular branches of the ascending pharyngeal artery's neuromeningeal trunk enter the skull base through the hypoglossal and jugular foramen, respectively. The jugular branch gives rise to a lateral clival branch, and the hypoglossal branch to a medial clival branch intracranially. Both the medial and lateral clival branches anastomose with the meningohypophyseal trunk and lateral clival artery. Through Jacobson's canal, the

inferior tympanic branch of the ascending pharyngeal artery connects with the caroticotypanic artery of the petrous ICA. In the middle ear, the inferior tympanic branch also anastomoses with multiple branches of the facial arcade: the superior tympanic artery, the mandibular branch of the ICA, the stylomastoid artery (which arises from the posterior auricular or occipital artery), the anterior tympanic artery of the proximal IMA, and the petrous branch of the MMA. Additionally, the marginal tentorial artery of Bernasconi and Cassanari (meningohypophyseal trunk) may anastomose with the posterior branch of the MMA. These connections are relevant to meningiomas arising from the tentorium cerebelli. Finally, the vidian artery, which arises from the distal IMA, travels through the vidian canal to the foramen lacerum. From there, it connects to the mandibular artery of the petrous ICA and has a classic horizontal appearance on

Cervicomedullary Region

Meningiomas located near the foramen magnum often are supplied by the occipital and ascending pharyngeal arteries. The vertebral artery, and the thyrocervical and costocervcial trunks of the sub-clavian artery, also provides vascular contribution. Multiple anastomotic connections between these extracranial vessels and the intracranial arteries place the cerebellum, occipital lobes, brainstem, lower cranial nerves, and spinal cord at risk during embolization.[2,34,37]

A very proximal musculospinal branch of the ascending pharyngeal artery anastomoses with the vertebral artery's C3 radicular anastomotic artery. The prevertebral branch is located more distally and usually arises from the neuromeningeal trunk, but can arise directly from the ascending pharyngeal artery. It connects to the vertebral artery via the C3 radicular anastomotic artery and the odontoid arch anteriorly along the C1 to C2 vertebra. This branch can be seen on lateral angiography as having a typical "U-shaped curve."[34,37,38] The occipital artery is a remnant of the types I and II proatlantal arteries, which serve as conduits in the late fetal stage between the carotid and vertebral systems. As a result, the occipital artery commonly has persistent connections to the vertebral arteries and may have connections to the carotid system. The stylomastoid artery often arises from the occipital artery (sometimes from the posterior auricular artery), contributing to the blood supply of the posterior fossa meninges. As a result, it can anastomose with the posterior meningeal branch of the vertebral artery (PMA) as well as the MMA, ascending pharyngeal, ILT, and the meningohypophseal trunk of the ECA and ICA.[34]

Cervical–medullary anastomoses connect the ascending cervical and posterior deep cervical artery branches of the thyrocervical trunk and cost-ocervical trunk, respectively, with the vertebral artery. On occasion, the vertebral artery can even arise directly from the thyrocervical trunk.[34]

Cranial Nerve Blood Supply

A summary of the cranial nerve blood supply can be found in **Table 2**. Excluding the potential loss of vision from inadvertent embolization of the OA or central retinal artery, the cranial nerves at highest risk are cranial nerve VII and the lower cranial nerves (IX-XII). There is a well-described arterial facial arcade that supplies the geniculate ganglion of cranial nerve VII. A precise understanding of the arterial supply to this arcade and its anatomic location is paramount to the interventionalist. The facial arcade typically arises at the connection between the petrous branch of the MMA and the sty-lomastoid branch of the posterior auricular artery (sometimes inclusive of the occipital artery). As previously noted, the neuromeningeal trunk of the ascending pharyngeal artery gives rise to the jugular and hypoglossal branches; these branches then traverse their named foramen through the skull base and provide arterial supply to the lower cranial nerves. Cranial nerves IX and XI derive their supply from the jugular branch, and cranial nerve XII from the hypoglossal branch (see **Table 2**). The more proximal, cisternal segments of these nerves are supplied by branches of the adjacent vertebral artery. The musculospinal artery branch of the ascending pharyngeal artery supplies cranial nerve XI. Distal embolization of these arteries with either liquid embolic agents or with particles smaller than 80 μm diameter can result in permanent injury to the associated cranial nerves. More proximal embolization may allow recovery of cranial nerve palsies with time and steroid therapy as collateral flow develops. One case report suggests that axonotmetic injury to the cranial nerves is possible during difficult removal of a microcatheter after liquid embolization. Delayed recovery was achieved in the reported case.[39]

COMPLICATIONS AND THEIR MANAGEMENT

Surgical morbidity associated with resection of large, vascularized meningiomas can be significant; however, the benefit of embolization is difficult to quantify and carries its own risks.[6,7] Proponents think that preoperative embolization offers decreased surgical morbidity in the setting of acceptably low complication rates. Opponents cite a lack of clinically significant benefit, and therefore consider even a very low complication rate unacceptable. Other critics acknowledge benefits of embolization, but suggest that complication rates are unacceptably high.

Reported complications associated with meningioma embolization include cerebral infarction owing to inadvertent embolization of uninvolved cerebral vessels, thromboembolism, periprocedural or postprocedural intracranial hemorrhage, tumor swelling with associated mass effect, infection,[40,41] and embolization to the pulmonary vasculature.[42] Hemorrhagic complications may occur owing to mechanical injury of the feeding artery by the microcatheter and wires, or upon catheter retrieval when using liquid embolic agents. Hemorrhagic complications are also thought to occur with greater frequency when substantial

Table 2
Summary of cranial nerve vascular supply

Cranial Nerve	Location	Intracranial Arterial Supply	Extracranial Arterial Supply
III	Cisternal	Mesencephalic perforators	—
	Cavernous	Inferior lateral trunk	
IV	Cavernous	Marginal artery of tentorium cerebelli, ILT, anteromedial branch of the ILT	—
V	Cisternal	Basilar vestige of trigeminal artery, SCA, AICA	—
	Meckel cave	Cavernous branch of MMA, ILT, Lateral artery of trigeminal ganglion	
V_2	Foramen rotundum	—	Artery of foramen rotundum from ILT
	Pterygopalatine fossa	—	Infraorbital artery
V_3	Foramen ovale	—	Posterior medial branch of the ILI
VII, VIII	Cistern + IAC	Labyrinthine artery	—
	Geniculate ganglion	—	Petrosal branch of MMA, stylomastoid branch of postauricular/occipital
IX	Cisternal, Jugular foramen	Jugular branch of neuromeningeal trunk	—
	Retrostyloid space	—	Ascending pharyngeal artery
	Tonsillar area	—	Descending palatine, sphenopalatine, ascending palatine, dorsal lingual
X	Cisternal, jugular foramen	Jugular branch of neuromeningeal trunk	—
XI	Spinal root	Anterior and posterior spinal	—
XII	Cisternal hypoglossal canal	Hypoglossal branch of neuromeningeal trunk	

Abbreviations: AICA, anterior inferior cerebellar artery; IAC, internal auditory canal; ILT, inferior lateral trunk; MMA, middle meningeal artery; SCA, superior cerebellar artery.

Data from Geibprasert S, Pongpech S, Armstrong D, et al. Dangerous extracranial-intracranial anastomoses and supply to the cranial nerves: vessels the neurointerventionalist needs to know. AJNR Am J Neuroradiol 2009;30(8):1459–68; and Hendrix P, Griessenauer CJ, Foreman P, et al. Arterial supply of the lower cranial nerves: a comprehensive review. Clin Anat 2014;27(1):108–17.

devascularization of the tumor results in significant tumor necrosis. This risk may be exacerbated when using very small particles or liquid embolic agents that penetrate deep into the tumor bed.[18] Other theories suggest that compromise of the tumor's venous outflow may increase the risk of hemorrhage in high-flow lesions.[2,43,44]

A recent literature review identified 36 reports published between 1990 and 2011 that included 459 patients who underwent meningioma embolization. Of these, 21 patients (4.6%) experienced complications related to embolization and 3 experienced a major complication or death (0.7%).[3] Several studies reported higher complication rates, although these were eliminated from the analysis owing to strict inclusion/exclusion criteria. One excluded study evaluated 167 patients with skull base meningiomas. The authors documented an immediate postembolization complication rate of 12.6%, with 9% of patients sustaining permanent injury. Recent larger series, using modern endovascular techniques, show a rate of symptomatic complications around 5%.[41,45,46]

Importantly, these complications must be compared with potential surgical morbidities in patients without embolization. These are difficult comparisons to make. High operative blood loss may be limited by anticipation, adjustments in surgical technique, and communication with anesthesiology. A prospective, randomized, controlled trial assessing surgical morbidity and mortality in patients treated with preoperative embolization may best answer these questions. However, such a study is difficult and expensive to undertake. Review of national quality databases or large, multicenter, prospective series may best inform future treatment paradigms.

POSTOPERATIVE CARE

Postoperatively, the patient should be awoken and a complete neurologic assessment performed. Patients should be observed in the intensive care unit or another closely monitored setting. In cases of large tumors, steroids are often beneficial to treat swelling after embolization. Delayed complications can include tumor edema, ischemia, and hemorrhage.[18,20]

OUTCOMES

The majority of studies comparing preoperative embolization to surgery without embolization are small, retrospective series. A nonrandomized, prospective study compared 30 patients who underwent preoperative embolization in 1 center with 30 patients from a second center who did not undergo embolization. Those patients with greater than 90% tumor embolization had decreased blood loss, but no other clearly identified benefit. No differences in surgical morbidity and mortality were demonstrated between the 2 groups.[11] A recent, larger series of 105 cases with 56 preoperative embolizations demonstrated a significant decrease in operative blood loss when adjusted for tumor volume. The comparison group, however, was historic.[41] A radiographic study, evaluating preembolization and postembolization tumor enhancement in 52 patients with meningiomas who underwent embolization and 37 who did not, showed no differences between groups. However, when adjusting for enhancement reduction on imaging, the group that underwent embolization exhibited less intraoperative blood loss and better postoperative outcomes, as defined by Karnofsky performance scores at 3 months.[46]

SUMMARY

Smaller meningiomas near the cortical surface with mild to moderate blood supply that exhibit low surgical risk most often do not require preoperative embolization. Meningiomas more likely to benefit from embolization are large convexity meningiomas with a vast arterial supply emanating from multiple sources in which profuse bleeding can be encountered with surgical removal of the bone flap.[3] Meningiomas at the skull base are more likely to benefit from embolization, but are more challenging to treat owing to potential complications related to embolic risk of dangerous anastomoses and cranial nerve injury. In rare situations, palliative embolization can be used effectively. The role for preoperative embolization of meningiomas remains unclear. The goals for embolization need to be discussed with the operative surgeon to best facilitate surgical benefit.

REFERENCES

1. Dowd CF, Halbach VV, Higashida RT. Meningiomas: the role of preoperative angiography and embolization. Neurosurg Focus 2003;15(1):E10.
2. Al-Mefty O, DeMonte F, McDermott MW. Al-Mefty's meningiomas. 2nd edition. New York: Thieme Medical; 2011.
3. Shah AH, Patel N, Raper DM, et al. The role of preoperative embolization for intracranial meningiomas. J Neurosurg 2013;119(2):364–72.
4. Nakamura M, Roser F, Michel J, et al. The natural history of incidental meningiomas. Neurosurgery 2003;53(1):62–70 [discussion: 70–1].
5. Yano S, Kuratsu J, Kumamoto Brain Tumor Research Group. Indications for surgery in patients with asymptomatic meningiomas based on an extensive experience. J Neurosurg 2006;105(4):538–43.
6. Chan RC, Thompson GB. Morbidity, mortality, and quality of life following surgery for intracranial meningiomas. A retrospective study in 257 cases. J Neurosurg 1984;60(1):52–60.
7. Awad IA, Kalfas I, Hahn JF, et al. Intracranial meningiomas in the aged: surgical outcome in the era of computed tomography. Neurosurgery 1989;24(4): 557–60.
8. Chun JY, McDermott MW, Lamborn KR, et al. Delayed surgical resection reduces intraoperative blood loss for embolized meningiomas. Neurosurgery 2002;50(6):1231–5 [discussion: 1235–7].
9. Brismar J, Cronqvist S. Therapeutic embolization in the external carotid artery region. Acta Radiol Diagn 1978;19(5):715–31.
10. Koike T, Sasaki O, Tanaka R, et al. Long-term results in a case of meningioma treated by embolization alone–case report. Neurol Med Chir 1990;30(3): 173–7.
11. Bendszus M, Rao G, Burger R, et al. Is there a benefit of preoperative meningioma embolization? Neurosurgery 2000;47(6):1306–11 [discussion: 1311–2].
12. Dubel GJ, Ahn SH, Soares GM. Contemporary endovascular embolotherapy for meningioma. Semin Intervent Radiol 2013;30(3):263–77.
13. Manelfe C, Lasjaunias P, Ruscalleda J. Preoperative embolization of intracranial meningiomas. AJNR Am J Neuroradiol 1986;7(5):963–72.

14. Shah A, Choudhri O, Jung H, et al. Preoperative endovascular embolization of meningiomas: update on therapeutic options. Neurosurg Focus 2015;38(3):E7.

15. Kai Y, Hamada J, Morioka M, et al. Appropriate interval between embolization and surgery in patients with meningioma. AJNR Am J Neuroradiol 2002; 23(1):139–42.

16. Nania A, Granata F, Vinci S, et al. Necrosis score, surgical time, and transfused blood volume in patients treated with preoperative embolization of intracranial meningiomas. Analysis of a single-centre experience and a review of literature. Clin Neuroradiol 2014;24(1):29–36.

17. Morris P. Interventional and endovascular therapy of the nervous system. New York: Springer-Verlag; 2002.

18. Carli DF, Sluzewski M, Beute GN, et al. Complications of particle embolization of meningiomas: frequency, risk factors, and outcome. AJNR Am J Neuroradiol 2010;31(1):152–4.

19. Wakhloo AK, Juengling FD, Van Volthoven V, et al. Extended preoperative polyvinyl alcohol microembolization of intracranial meningiomas: assessment of two embolization techniques. AJNR Am J Neuroradiol 1993;14(3):571–82.

20. Bendszus M, Monoranu CM, Schutz A, et al. Neurologic complications after particle embolization of intracranial meningiomas. AJNR Am J Neuroradiol 2005;26(6):1413–9.

21. Hamada J, Ushio Y, Kazekawa K, et al. Embolization with cellulose porous beads, I: an experimental study. AJNR Am J Neuroradiol 1996; 17(10):1895–9.

22. Kai Y, Hamada JI, Morioka M, et al. Clinical evaluation of cellulose porous beads for the therapeutic embolization of meningiomas. AJNR Am J Neuroradiol 2006;27(5):1146–50.

23. Bendszus M, Klein R, Burger R, et al. Efficacy of trisacryl gelatin microspheres versus polyvinyl alcohol particles in the preoperative embolization of meningiomas. AJNR Am J Neuroradiol 2000;21(2):255–61.

24. Kim LJ, Albuquerque FC, Aziz-Sultan A, et al. Low morbidity associated with use of n-butyl cyanoacrylate liquid adhesive for preoperative transarterial embolization of central nervous system tumors. Neurosurgery 2006;59(1):98–104 [discussion: 98–104].

25. Gobin YP, Murayama Y, Milanese K, et al. Head and neck hypervascular lesions: embolization with ethylene vinyl alcohol copolymer–laboratory evaluation in Swine and clinical evaluation in humans. Radiology 2001;221(2):309–17.

26. Shi ZS, Feng L, Jiang XB, et al. Therapeutic embolization of meningiomas with Onyx for delayed surgical resection. Surg Neurol 2008;70(5):478–81.

27. Feng L, Kienitz BA, Matsumoto C, et al. Feasibility of using hyperosmolar mannitol as a liquid tumor embolization agent. AJNR Am J Neuroradiol 2005; 26(6):1405–12.

28. Jungreis CA. Skull-base tumors: ethanol embolization of the cavernous carotid artery. Radiology 1991;181(3):741–3.

29. Kubo M, Kuwayama N, Hirashima Y, et al. Hydroxyapatite ceramics as a particulate embolic material: report of the clinical experience. AJNR Am J Neuroradiol 2003;24(8):1545–7.

30. Kubo M, Kuwayama N, Hirashima Y, et al. Hydroxyapatite ceramics as a particulate embolic material: report of the physical properties of the hydroxyapatite particles and the animal study. AJNR Am J Neuroradiol 2003;24(8):1540–4.

31. Probst EN, Grzyska U, Westphal M, et al. Preoperative embolization of intracranial meningiomas with a fibrin glue preparation. AJNR Am J Neuroradiol 1999;20(9):1695–702.

32. Yasui K, Shoda Y, Suyama T, et al. Preoperative embolization for meningioma using lipiodol. Interv Neuroradiol 1998;4(Suppl 1):63–6.

33. Perrini P, Cardia A, Fraser K, et al. A microsurgical study of the anatomy and course of the ophthalmic artery and its possibly dangerous anastomoses. J Neurosurg 2007;106(1):142–50.

34. Geibprasert S, Pongpech S, Armstrong D, et al. Dangerous extracranial-intracranial anastomoses and supply to the cranial nerves: vessels the neurointerventionalist needs to know. AJNR Am J Neuroradiol 2009;30(8):1459–68.

35. Lasjaunias P, Moret J, Mink J. The anatomy of the inferolateral trunk (ILT) of the internal carotid artery. Neuroradiology 1977;13(4):215–20.

36. Tubbs RS, Hansasuta A, Loukas M, et al. Branches of the petrous and cavernous segments of the internal carotid artery. Clin Anat 2007;20(6):596–601.

37. Hacein-Bey L, Daniels DL, Ulmer JL, et al. The ascending pharyngeal artery: branches, anastomoses, and clinical significance. AJNR Am J Neuroradiol 2002;23(7):1246–56.

38. Haffajee MR. A contribution by the ascending pharyngeal artery to the arterial supply of the odontoid process of the axis vertebra. Clin Anat 1997; 10(1):14–8.

39. Nyberg EM, Chaudry MI, Turk AS, et al. Transient cranial neuropathies as sequelae of Onyx embolization of arteriovenous shunt lesions near the skull base: possible axonotmetic traction injuries. J Neurointerv Surg 2013;5(4):e21.

40. Yen PS, Lin CC, Lee CC, et al. CNS Clostridium perfringens infection: a rare complication of preoperative embolization of meningioma. AJNR Am J Neuroradiol 2006;27(6):1355–6.

41. Ishihara H, Ishihara S, Niimi J, et al. The safety and efficacy of preoperative embolization of meningioma with N-butyl cyanoacrylate. Interv Neuroradiol 2015; 21(5):624–30.

42. Pelz DM, Lownie SP, Fox AJ, et al. Symptomatic pulmonary complications from liquid acrylate embolization of brain arteriovenous malformations. AJNR Am J Neuroradiol 1995;16(1):19–26.

43. Kallmes DF, Evans AJ, Kaptain GJ, et al. Hemorrhagic complications in embolization of a meningioma: case report and review of the literature. Neuroradiology 1997;39(12):877–80.

44. Yu SC, Boet R, Wong GK, et al. Postembolization hemorrhage of a large and necrotic meningioma. AJNR Am J Neuroradiol 2004; 25(3):506–8.

45. Aihara M, Naito I, Shimizu T, et al. Preoperative embolization of intracranial meningiomas using n-butyl cyanoacrylate. Neuroradiology 2015;57(7): 713–9.

46. Ali R, Khan M, Chang V, et al. MRI pre- and post-embolization enhancement patterns predict surgical outcomes in intracranial meningiomas. J Neuroimaging 2015. [Epub ahead of print].

Genomic and Epigenomic Landscape in Meningioma

Wenya Linda Bi, MD, PhD[a,b], Yu Mei, MD, PhD[a], Pankaj K. Agarwalla, MD[b],
Rameen Beroukhim, MD, PhD[b], Ian F. Dunn, MD[a,*]

KEYWORDS

- Meningioma • Genomics • Epigenetics • Molecular taxonomy • Precision medicine

KEY POINTS

- The natural history of meningiomas is incompletely predicted by their histopathologic grade and treatment history.
- Recurrent somatic mutations in *NF2*, *TRAF7*, *KLF4*, *AKT1*, and *SMO* are collectively present in approximately 80% of sporadic meningiomas, as identified by next-generation sequencing.
- Epigenetic alterations, particularly methylation changes, influence the transcriptional accessibility and consequent expression of a gene, without change in the DNA sequence.
- Epigenetic alterations serve as a complementary strategy for biologic modulation of targeted therapies in meningioma.

INTRODUCTION

Meningiomas are the most common primary intracranial neoplasms in adults, accounting for 35.8% of all primary central nervous system (CNS) tumors and more than 53% of all benign CNS tumors diagnosed in the United States.[1] The majority of meningiomas are considered benign,[2] although a small proportion display malignant behavior characterized by invasive growth patterns and/or markedly higher recurrence rates. These are classified by the World Health Organization as grades I, II, and III, with higher grades associated with significantly greater rates of morbidity and mortality despite aggressive multimodality treatment.[3]

Patients with grade I, or benign, meningiomas have a 10-year overall survival rate of 80% and a progression-free survival rate of approximately 74% to 96%, which is dependent on treatment modality, extent of resection, location of tumor, and likely age.[4–6] Grade II meningiomas are associated with up to 8-fold greater recurrence rates than grade I meningiomas, with a 10-year overall survival of 53% to 79% and progression-free survival of 23% to 78%, depending on the extent of resection and adjuvant therapies.[7–10] Grade III meningiomas are associated with a 10-year overall survival rate of 14% to 34% and progression-free survival rate of 0%.[8,11]

Although histologic grade serves as a powerful tool in prognostication of the natural history, it inconsistently predicts biologic behavior; meningiomas with benign histologic features can recur at significant rates despite aggressive resection, whereas meningiomas with high-grade features respond variably to adjuvant treatment, such as radiation. Attempts to further stratify meningiomas into histologic subtypes within each grade also fail to enhance predictive value for patient outcomes consistently. In recent decades, a paradigm shift toward molecular taxonomy has transformed the management of several tumor types. Within the

Disclosure Statement: All authors contributed to this article and attest to no conflicts of interest. All authors have no financial disclosures.

[a] Department of Neurosurgery, Brigham and Women's Hospital, Harvard Medical School, 15 Francis Street, PBB-3, Boston, MA, USA; [b] Department of Cancer Biology, Dana-Farber Cancer Institute, Harvard Medical School, Boston, MA, USA

* Corresponding author. Department of Neurosurgery, Brigham and Women's Hospital, 15 Francis Street, Boston, MA 02115.

E-mail address: idunn@partners.org

neurosurgery.theclinics.com

CNS, medulloblastomas, glioblastomas, and ependymomas provide benchmarks for integrating molecular diagnoses with clinical decision making for adjuvant treatment and predicting clinical course.[12–14] Recent advances in meningioma genomics and epigenomics have yielded greater understanding of their biology and provide an initial framework for their molecular stratification. This review highlights contemporary concepts in the genomics and epigenomics of intracranial meningiomas and their applications in diagnosis, prognosis, and management.

GENOMICS AND EPIGENOMICS IN MENINGIOMA

Genomic alterations encompass mutations, insertions, deletions, and rearrangements across the genome. Elucidation of critical oncogenic drivers in a number of cancers (eg, BRAF in melanoma[15] or cKIT in gastrointestinal stromal tumors and chronic myelogenous leukemia[16]) has enabled targeted therapies in the so-called mutation-to-drug paradigm. Such approaches have not been possible in meningioma until recently, when unbiased genome- and exome-wide sequencing approaches have implicated a central core of genetic mutations that are associated with a substantial percentage of meningiomas.[17,18] These alterations have highlighted an association between genotype and phenotype in meningiomas, and have suggested potential targets for pharmacotherapeutics.

However, approximately 20% of meningiomas do not have an identifiable oncogenic driver mutation to date.[19] In these, as well as other meningiomas, epigenomic alterations may play a significant role in tumor development and progression.[20] Epigenomic modifications include DNA nucleotide methylation, microRNA interactions, histone packaging, and chromatin restructuring, all of which alter the transcriptional accessibility of the primary genetic script without change in the actual gene sequence.[21] Of these, methylation has been the most extensively studied, with approximately 77% of meningiomas harboring at least 1 methylated gene and 25% with 3 or more such alterations.[22] Notably, the ability of cells to introduce and reverse epigenetic modifications affords additional opportunity for fine modulation and targeted inhibition of tumor growth.[23]

Just as an improved understanding of genomic and epigenomic alterations has changed the classification and treatment of cancers such as chronic myelogenous leukemia, lymphomas, melanoma, and lung cancer, similar interrogation of the meningioma genome and epigenome hold significant promise for novel clinical trials for patients harboring these tumors.[24,25]

Genetic Alterations

Initial insight into the genetic alterations that lead to meningiomas was derived from associated familial syndromes. The first and most thoroughly described of these syndromes is neurofibromatosis 2 (NF2), in which 50% to 75% of patients develop 1 or more meningiomas. The underlying gene, NF2, is a well-defined tumor suppressor that encodes the protein Merlin. Mutation, allelic inactivation, or loss of the tumor suppressor NF2 gene and its parent chromosome 22 have been implicated in approximately 40% to 60% of sporadic meningiomas in addition to those afflicted with neurofibromatosis.[17,18,26,27] NF2 likely plays an early driver role in meningioma formation, given its alteration in both low-grade and high-grade tumors,[28] as well as the development of meningiomas in NF2 knockout mice.[29,30]

In addition, the recent application of next-generation DNA sequencing approaches has identified recurrent somatic mutations in 4 genes that collectively are present in approximately 40% of sporadic meningiomas, usually without associated NF2 mutation or chromosome 22 loss (**Fig. 1**).[17,18] These genes are the proapoptotic E3 ubiquitin ligase TNF receptor-associated factor 7 (TRAF7), the pluripotency transcription factor Kruppel-like factor 4 (KLF4), the protooncogene v-Akt murine thymoma viral oncogene homolog 1 (AKT1), and the Hedgehog pathway signaling member smoothened (SMO).

Mutations in TRAF7, located on chromosome 16p13, are observed in 12% to 25% of meningiomas.[18] A majority of meningiomas with TRAF7 mutations also harbor mutations in KLF4 or AKT1 mutations, but not both.[18,31] In contrast, TRAF7 mutations rarely co-occur with SMO mutations, NF2 mutations, or chromosome 22 loss.[18] The mechanism and downstream effectors of this mutation remain to be elucidated.

Approximately 15% of grade I meningiomas possess a recurrent mutation in the transcription factor gene KLF4, located on chromosome 9q31, with a resultant lysine to glutamine substitution at codon 409 (K409Q). KLF4 mutations co-occur with TRAF7 mutations and are exclusive of NF2 and AKT1 mutations.[18] During development, KLF4 promotes reprogramming of differentiated somatic cells back to a pluripotent state.[32] Alteration of this pluripotent transcription factor may represent a recapitulation of embryologic mechanisms to drive tumor formation.

Another 6.8% of meningiomas harbor a recurrent mutation in AKT1, located on chromosome 14q32,

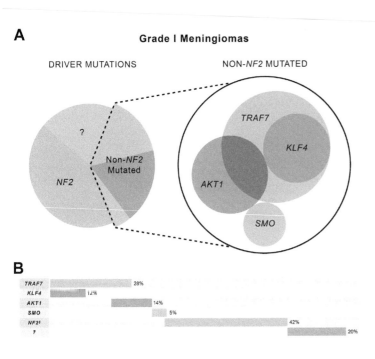

A

Grade I Meningiomas

DRIVER MUTATIONS   NON-*NF2* MUTATED

?

Non-*NF2*
Mutated

NF2

TRAF7

KLF4

AKT1

SMO

B

TRAF7	28%
KLF4	12%
AKT1	14%
SMO	5%
NF2[a]	42%
?	20%

Fig. 1. Distribution of NF2, AKT1, SMO, TRAF7, and KLF4 mutations in grade I meningiomas. (*A*) Recurrent oncogenic driver mutations in grade I meningiomas include *TRAF7*, *AKT1*, *KLF4*, and *SMO*, which largely occur in a mutually exclusive pattern with *NF2*. Mutations in *KLF4* and *AKT1* overlap with *TRAF7*, in proportion to the areas represented in the Venn diagram. (*B*) Distribution of *TRAF7*, *AKT1*, *KLF4*, *SMO*, and *NF2* mutations across grade I meningiomas. Recurrent oncogenic changes remain unclear for approximately 20% of meningiomas (designated by ?). [a] *NF2* mutation or loss. (*Data from* Refs.[17–19])

which produces a known oncogenic alteration of glutamic acid to lysine at codon 17 (E17K).[18,33] These occur in conjunction with *TRAF7* mutations in a subpopulation of meningiomas, but remain exclusive of *NF2*, *KLF4*, and *SMO* mutations.[18] *AKT1*[E17K] mutation results in activation of downstream effectors of the *PI3K/AKT/mTOR* oncogenic pathway, rendering it a potential target by selective AKT inhibitors, several of which are currently in phase I and II clinical testing for the treatment of a broad range of cancers, including carcinoma of the breast, lung, and colon.[34]

Last, approximately 5.5% of grade I meningiomas, or greater than 10% of non–*NF2*-altered tumors, express mutations in *SMO*.[17,18] These *SMO* alterations result in downstream activation of Hedgehog signaling, another well-characterized pathway in cancer that is notably dysregulated in basal cell carcinoma and medulloblastoma.[35,36] In basal cell carcinoma, where more than 90% of tumors have mutations in either *SMO* or *PTCH*, inhibition of SMO has been particularly effective in the setting of locally advanced or metastatic disease, with vismodegib receiving approval from the US Food and Drug Administration in 2012.[37] Clinical trials testing SMO inhibitors for recurrent meningiomas with *SMO* mutations are now underway.

Chromosomal Copy Number Alterations

In addition to changes at the single nucleotide level, meningiomas harbor a classic array of chromosomal copy number alterations, especially in higher grade tumors. The most commonly observed chromosomal change is monosomy of chromosome 22, observed in in 40% to 70% of meningiomas.[38] Aside from monosomy 22, the copy number landscape of benign meningiomas is typically neutral. One exception is the angiomatous subtype of grade I meningiomas, which characteristically express multiple polysomies across the genome, most commonly of chromosome 5.[30]

As meningiomas progress to a higher grade state, an increasing number of chromosomal gains and losses are observed. In atypical and anaplastic meningiomas, these include frequent loss of chromosome 1p, 6q, 10, 14q, and 18q, as well as gain of chromosomes 1q, 9q, 12q, 15q, 17q, and 20q (**Fig. 2**).[38,40,41] Among these, chromosome 1p and 14q loss are the most frequent cytogenetic abnormality observed in meningiomas after chromosome 22, affecting one-half of grade II and nearly all grade III meningiomas.[40] Investigations into candidate oncogenes on these chromosomal arms have yet to elucidate clear drivers in meningioma tumorigenesis.

Epigenetic Alterations

Beyond structural and genomic aberrations, an array of gene expression studies have implicated a role for epigenetic silencing of genes in the absence of inactivating mutations.[22,42–44] Identification of somatic mutations in the chromatin remodeling complex gene *SMARCB1* and the

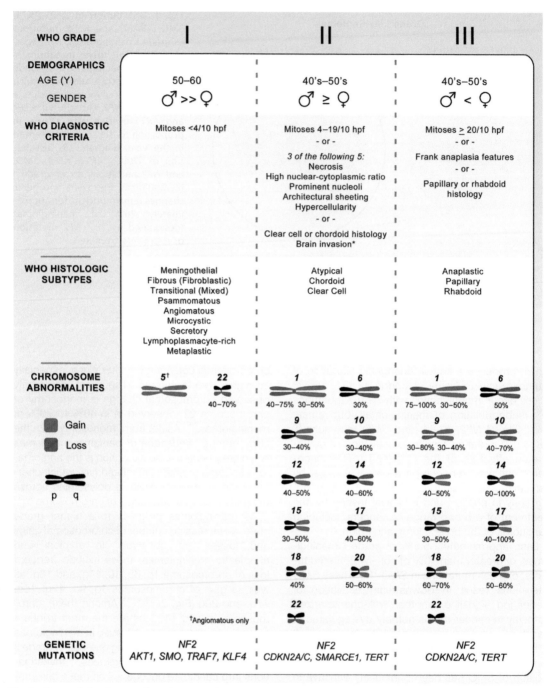

Fig. 2. Genomic landscape of grade I, II, and III meningiomas. Demographics, current World Health Organization diagnostic criteria, histologic subtypes, recurrent copy number alterations, and mutations across meningiomas. (*From* Bi WL, Abedalthagafi M, Horowitz P, et al. Genomic landscape of intracranial meningiomas. J Neurosurg. Published online January 15, 2016; http://dx.doi.org/10.3171/2015.6.JNS15591.)

histone demethylases *KDM5C* and *KDM6A* in meningiomas further supports a role for epigenetic modification driving tumor inception.[17]

To date, a large number of epigenetic markers have been associated with meningioma

tumorigenesis (**Table 1**). Many epigenetic loci associated with meningioma are associated with the early stages of signaling pathways related to cell proliferation or apoptosis, making them important targets for successful interruption of

Table 1
Epigenetic modifications implicated in meningioma tumorigenesis

Gene	Product: Normal Function	Epigenetic Change	Association of Change in Meningioma
CDKN2A[44]	p14ARF protein: TP53 and cell cycle regulator (tumor suppressor)	Hypermethylation	Tumorigenesis
TP73[74]	p73: cell growth and cell cycle arrest regulation (tumor suppressor)	Hypermethylation	Tumorigenesis
MEG3[75]	Noncoding RNA: p53 activation activity (tumor suppressor)	Hypermethylation	Tumorigenesis
HOXA5, HOXA6, HOXA9, HOXA11[53]	HOXA5, HOXA6, HOXA9, HOXA11	Comethylation	Tumorigenesis
IGF2BP1[53]	RNA binding protein: mRNA stability and translocation regulation	Hypermethylation	Tumorigenesis
WNK2[55]	Serine–threonine kinase: negative regulation of epidermal growth factor receptor signaling (cell signaling)	Hypermethylation	Tumorigenesis
LMO4[76]	LIM domain transcription factor LMO4: TGF-β signal modulator (cell signaling)	Downregulation	Tumorigenesis
HES1[77,78]	Hairy and enhancer of split-1 family bHLH transcription factor 1: Notch signaling activation (cell signaling)	Upregulation	Tumorigenesis
MGMT[79]	O6-alkylguanine DNA alkyltransferase: DNA repair	Methylation	Tumorigenesis
miR-200a[80]	micro-RNA: E-cadherin upregulation	Downregulation	Tumorigenesis
UPK3A[53]	Uroplakin-3a transmembrane protein: cytoskeleton regulation	Hypermethylation	Growth factor
PENK[53]	Preproenkephalin: p53 interaction for stress-induced apoptosis	Hypermethylation	Apoptosis
THBS1[81]	Thrombospondin 1: angiogenesis inhibition	Methylation	Angiogenesis
HIF3α[53,82]	Hypoxia inducible factor 3, alpha subunit: dominant negative regulator of HIF-1alpha	Methylation	Angiogenesis

Abbreviation: TGF, transforming growth factor.
  Data from Refs.[44,53,55,76–82]

uncontrolled tumor growth. In vitro and in vivo efforts have largely focused on controlling the outcomes of aberrant DNA methylation, of which hypermethylation generally results in transcriptional gene silencing and, conversely, hypomethylation leads to gene activation.

Because hypermethylation commonly produces an inhibitory effect, recovery of the associated tumor-suppressing activity represent one therapeutic strategy. As an example, aberrant histone methylation of the retinoblastoma zinc-finger (*RIZ1*) methyltransferase gene is associated with cell cycle deregulation in a number of tumors.[45–48] Normal RIZ1 activity halts cell proliferation at the G2-M cell phase and encourages apoptosis through downregulation of c-Myc and thioredoxin binding protein.[49] In meningioma, RIZ1 expression negatively correlates with tumor grade, with grade I, II, and III meningiomas expressing RIZ1 in 87.5%, 38.9%, and 23.8% of cases, respectively. Replacement of RIZ1 expression with a transactivating fusion protein resulted in decreased cell proliferation in primary meningioma cells and reduced meningioma burden in xenograft mouse models.[50]

Conversely, therapies that interrupt the inhibitory hypermethylation effect on tumor suppressors can also address downstream prooncogenic pathways. Comethylation of several homeobox (HOX) genes, which are well-known to contribute to normal organ development and function, has also been implicated in the tumorigenesis of high-grade meningiomas.[51–53] Concordant silencing of HOXA genes on chromosome 7p15.2 occurs with HOXA5, HOXA6, HOXA9, and HOXA11. HOXA9 has since been studied more extensively given its suggested role in malignant transformation, perhaps through protooncogene activation of Erg, Flt3, Lmo2, Myb, and Sox4.[53,54] Despite the functional redundancies across the many known HOX genes, a cytostatic peptide inhibitor (HXR9) that disrupts the interaction between HOXA9 and its cofactor, PBX, reduces cell line proliferation and tumor size in heterotopic mouse models.

The identification of aberrantly hypermethylated genes also allows application of existing demethylation agents in therapeutic trials. One example is the use of 5-aza-2'-deoxycytidine, an pharmacologic methylation inhibitor approved by the US Food and Drug Administration, on the kinase tumor suppressor, WNK2.[25,55] WNK2 negatively regulates MEK1/ERK1/2 and epidermal growth factor receptor signaling to inhibit subsequent cell proliferation and tumor colony formation.[56] Aberrant hypermethylation of WNK2 at it 5′ CpG island promotor, a stereotypical site of methylation events, is associated with 83% and 71% of grade II and III meningioma, among other brain tumors.[55,57] Some cell lines treated with 5-aza-2'-deoxycytidine could successfully reactivate WNK2 and decreased colony forming units. Although such in vitro models are far from clinical application, increased understanding of the potential and limits of epigenetic modulation serves as a powerful adjunct in the treatment of challenging tumors.

MOLECULAR TAXONOMY IN MENINGIOMA

The surge in genomic and epigenomic data on meningiomas has allowed increasing appreciation of associations between molecular signatures with characteristic phenotypes, intracranial locations, and tumor grade.

Genetic Hallmarks of Meningioma Subtypes

Inactivation of NF2 has long been observed to occur in 70% to 80% of fibroblastic and transitional meningiomas but less than 1% of secretory meningiomas. This striking difference in mutation frequency suggests that some morphologic subtypes of meningioma harbor subtype-specific oncogenic mutations other than NF2, which was corroborated by the discovery of mutations in TRAF7, KLF4, AKT1, and SMO (Table 2).

Nearly all cases of secretory meningioma harbor mutations in both TRAF7 and KLF4^{K409Q} but lack mutations in NF2.[31] In particular, the KLF4 mutation has not been observed in nonsecretory meningiomas, CNS tumors, or other systemic malignancies. TRAF7 mutations overlap with KLF4 mutations, but are found in a larger spectrum of meningioma subtypes,[18] including 97% of secretory meningiomas and 8% of nonsecretory meningiomas.[31] AKT1 mutations, in contrast, are common in meningothelial meningiomas but increasingly rare with progressively higher grades of malignancy.[33] Additionally, clear cell meningiomas, in the hereditary multiple spinal meningioma syndrome and some cranial locations, are associated with loss-of-function mutations in SMARCE1.[58,59]

Specific genetic alterations not only associate with histopathologic subtype, they also correlate with anatomic location of tumors. Convexity meningiomas more often harbor mutations in NF2 and chromosome 22 loss of heterozygosity, and belong to the fibroblastic and transitional subtypes. In contrast, meningiomas along the anterior

Table 2 Meningioma subtype specific genetic alterations		
Subtype	Associated Genetic Alteration	Inheritance
Meningothelial	AKT (E17K)	Sporadic
Fibroblastic, transitional	NF2	Sporadic, Familial
Secretory	KLF4 (K409Q), TRAF7	Sporadic
Angiomatous	Polysomy 5	Sporadic
Clear cell	SMARCE1	Familial
Chordoid	der (1) t (1;3) (p12–13;q11) translocation	Sporadic

cranial base are more likely to express mutations in *SMO* or *AKT1/TRAF7*, with preserved chromosome 22q.[17,18] This corroborates with observations that cranial base meningiomas are predominantly of the meningothelial subtype, because *AKT1* mutations are largely found in meningothelial meningiomas.[17,60]

Epigenetic Stratification of Meningiomas

Epigenetic alterations have also been extensively scrutinized as potential biomarkers in meningioma grade and propensity to progress.[57] Evidence suggests that methylation often influences the early stages of oncogenesis and that epigenetic changes may require a critical threshold before influencing the phenotype of a tumor. Therefore, epigenetic changes may serve as an early harbinger to signal malignant transformation and suppression of such modifications may curtail recurrence in a more aggressive form.

However, the pattern of epigenetic modification varies widely among genes and observation of hypermethylation does not necessarily translate to suppressed transcription, or conversely for hypomethylated genes (**Table 3**). For example, whereas *ADCY3*, *GAS7*, *LAG3*, *LRR32*, and *SPON2* hypomethylation are more prominent in malignant meningiomas,[57] hypermethylation of *HOXA7*, *HOXA9*, and *HOXA10* are associated with high-grade meningiomas.[61]

Despite such heterogeneity in the epigenomic literature, several candidates have garnered interest in helping to differentiate grades II and III meningioma (see **Table 3**). One such marker of high-grade meningioma is tissue inhibitor of metalloproteinase 3 (*TIMP3*). Hypermethylation of *TIMP3* on chromosome 22q12 is observed in 67% of grade III meningiomas, compared with 17% of grade I and 22% of grade II meningiomas.[22,44,53,62] Hypermethylation of *NDRG2* and *MAL2*, leading to loss of expression, have also been correlated with malignant meningioma but not benign ones.[43,57] In comparison, hypermethylation of *TP73*, a functional homolog of *TP53*, seems to be increased in lower grade tumors after controlling for 1p chromosomal deletion.[42,63] Taken together, the complex array of epigenetic modifications leading to altered gene expression likely synergizes with concomitant genetic mutations and chromosomal alterations during oncogenesis of a malignant meningioma.[64,65]

MOLECULAR PREDICTORS OF CLINICAL OUTCOME

Aside from the role of molecular biomarkers in abetting the diagnosis of meningioma, a fundamental question in the clinical management of meningioma patients is the risk of recurrence after surgical resection. This poses a particular quandary among grade II meningiomas, for which no consensus exists regarding appropriate adjuvant treatment modality and timing. Recently, analysis of a cohort of atypical meningiomas after gross total resection revealed an association between increased chromosomal copy number alterations and risk of recurrence.[66] By summing the incidence of broad copy number events across an aggregate pool of common chromosomal aberrations in meningiomas, this strategy bypasses the limitations of assessing isolated molecular candidates in meningioma oncogenesis and offers a rapid molecular appraisal of potential outcome through routine clinical cytogenetic testing. In other words, patients harboring grade II meningiomas with high chromosomal disruption, which may have a greater risk of recurrence, may benefit from closer surveillance or adjuvant therapies.

Multiple gains and losses of chromosomal arms may reflect a more pervasive underlying genomic instability, resulting from the convergence of several aberrant signaling pathways. Another innate source of genomic instability relates to progressive lengthening of telomeres.[67-71] Telomerase activation has been demonstrated in 10% of grade I, 50% of grade II, and 95% of grade III meningiomas. Interestingly, mutations of the telomerase reverse transcriptase (*TERT*) gene promoter, and resultant increased expression of *TERT* mRNA, are associated with meningioma that relapse, with the highest frequency of *TERT* promoter mutations (28%) present in recurrent meningioma that have undergone histologic progression.[72]

Epigenetic alterations of single genes as well as panels of genes have also been associated with meningioma recurrence (**Table 4**). Notably, a scoring system based on quantified methylation values of 5 genes (*HOXA6*, *HOXA9*, *PENK*, *UPK3A*, and *IGF2bP1*), was reported to provide 80% to 90% sensitivity and specificity in predicting recurrence of meningiomas, independent of tumor grade.[53] Likewise, a microRNA signature of meningiomas recurrence has been recently reported,[73] with increased expression of miR-190a and miR-96-5p and downregulation of miR-29c-3p and miR-219-5p associated with high recurrence rates.

The validity of all such molecular prognostication strategies remains to be proven in future studies. If corroborated, they may serve a powerful tool in counseling patients, guiding management decisions, and stratifying clinical trials.

Table 3
Epigenetic modifications with diagnostic implications in meningioma

Genes with Diagnostic Implications	Product: Normal Function	Epigenetic Change	Association of Change in Meningioma
IGF2BP1[83]	RNA binding protein: mRNA stability and translocation regulation	Methylation	Malignant Potential
PDCD1[83]	Programmed cell death 1 protein: preventing immune cell targeting	Methylation	Malignant Potential
MAL2[57]	Mal proteolipid protein 2: membrane protein with potential role in apoptosis	Hypermethylation	Higher grade
TIMP3[22]	Metalloproteinase inhibitor 3: tumor suppressor	Hypermethylation	Higher grade
uPA[84,85]	Urokinase plasminogen activator: extracellular membrane proteolysis facilitating adhesion and migration, tumor suppressor	Hypomethylation	Higher grade
MEG3[75]	Noncoding RNA: p53 activation activity, tumor suppressor	Hypermethylation	Higher grade
NDRG2[43]	N-Nyc downstream regulated gene 2 protein: regulation of cell growth and apoptosis, cell signaling	Hypermethylation	Grade 3
IGF2, IGFBP2, IGFBP3, IGF2BP2[86,87]	IGF pathway protein and binding proteins: cellular proliferation and apoptosis inhibition, cell signaling	Upregulation	Grade 3
WNK2[55]	Serine–threonine kinase: negative regulation of epidermal growth factor receptor signaling, cell signaling	Hypermethylation	Grade 1 <2/3
TP73[63]	p73: cell growth and cell cycle arrest regulation, tumor suppressor	Hypermethylation	Grade 1 <2/3
GSTP1	Glutathione S transferase 1: conjugation of carcinogens to glutathione for detoxification, tumor suppressor	Hypermethylation	Grade 1 <2 <3
HOXA7, HOXA9, HOXA10[61]	Homeobox A gene cluster: determination of cellular identity and nervous system development, cell signaling	Comethylation	Grade 1 <2 <3
KDM5C[17]	Histone demethylase: chromatin structuring	Chromatin deregulation secondary to mutation	Grade 1 and 3
KDM6A[17]	Histone demethylase: chromatin structuring	Chromatin deregulation secondary to mutation	Grade 2
SMARCB1[17,58]	Chromatin remodeling complex protein: chromatin structuring	Chromatin deregulation secondary to mutation	Grade 1
miR-29c-3p[73]	microRNA: proliferation control	Downregulation	Grade 1 >2 >3
miR-219-5p[73]	microRNA: proliferation control and induction of apoptosis	Downregulation	Grade 1 >2 >3
miR-190a[73]	microRNA: antiapoptosis	Upregulation	Grade 1 <2 <3
Global[57] Hypomethylation	Increased expression of ADCY3, GAS7, LAG3, LRR32 and SPON2 without statistical significance	Hypomethylation	Higher grade

Abbreviations: IGF, insulinlike growth factor; mRNA, messenger RNA.
Data from Refs.[17,22,43,55,57,58,61,63,73,75,83–87]

Table 4
Epigenetic modifications with prognostic implications in meningioma

Genes with Prognostic Implications	Product: Normal Function	Epigenetic Change	Association of Change in Meningioma
IGF2, IGFBP2[88]	Insulin-like growth factor binding protein 2: cellular proliferation and apoptosis inhibition (cell signaling)	Upregulation	Tumor aggressiveness
NDRG2[43]	N-Myc downstream regulated gene 2 protein: regulation of cell growth and apoptosis (cell signaling)	Hypermethylation	Tumor aggressiveness
uPA[84,85]	Urokinase plasminogen activator: extracellular membrane proteolysis facilitating adhesion and migration (tumor suppressor)	Hypomethylation	Tumor aggressiveness
RASSF1A[63]	Ras-association domain family 1 protein: regulation of apoptosis and cell cycle progression	Hypermethylation	Malignant transformation
TP73[63]	p73: cell growth and cell cycle arrest regulation (tumor suppressor)	Hypermethylation	Malignant transformation
MAL2[57]	Mal proteolipid protein 2: membrane protein with potential role in apoptosis	Hypermethylation	Malignant transformation
miR-145[89]	microRNA: collagen regulation	Upregulation	Reduced proliferation, increased sensitivity to apoptosis, impaired migration
TMEM30B[90]	Transmembrane factor: cell cycle control (tumor suppressor)	Hypermethylation	Recurrence
HIST1H1C[91]	Histone H1.2: maintenance of methylation of pattern (tumor suppressor)	Upregulation	Recurrence
SFPR1[91]	Frizzled-related protein: Wnt downregulation (cell signaling)	Hypermethylation	Recurrence
LMO4[91]	LIM domain transcription factor LMO4: TGF-β signal modulator (cell signaling)	Downregulation	Primary (vs recurrent) meningioma
TIMP3[92]	Metalloproteinase inhibitor 3 (tumor suppressor)	Hypermethylation	Earlier recurrence

(continued on next page)

Table 4
(continued)

Genes with Prognostic Implications	Product: Normal Function	Epigenetic Change	Association of Change in Meningioma
miR-29c-3p[73]	microRNA: proliferation control	Upregulation	Higher recurrence
miR-219-5p[73]	microRNA: proliferation control and induction of apoptosis	Upregulation	Higher recurrence
miR-190a[73]	microRNA: anti-apoptosis	Upregulation	Higher recurrence
miR-96-5p[73]	microRNA: downregulation of cell cycle control and cell death	Upregulation	Higher recurrence
miR-190a, miR-29c-3p, miR-219-5p, miR-17-5p, miR-22-3p, miR-24-3p, miR-26b-5p, miR-27a-3p, miR-27b-3p, miR-96-5p, miR-146a-5p, miR-155-5p, miR-186-5p, 199a[73]	microRNA signature	—	Recurrence
HOXA6, HOXA9, PENK, UPK3A, IGF2BP1[53]	Epigenetically modified genes in prognostic scoring system	—	Recurrence

Abbreviation: TGF, transforming growth factor.
Data from Refs.[43,53,57,63,73,84,85,88,90–92]

SUMMARY

The application of large-scale molecular, genomic, and epigenetic profiling has ushered in a renaissance in the study of meningiomas. These systematic approaches inform a molecular taxonomy that promises to influence diagnosis, disease classification, and, ultimately, clinical management. Indeed, the mutational, copy number, and gene expression profiles of meningiomas are increasingly appreciated to predict histologic phenotype and clinical outcome, offering profound implications for adjuvant therapy options and patient counseling.

A further understanding of the factors that drive meningioma development and progression may lead to the classification of every patient's tumor according to its signature alterations, ushering in an era in which meningiomas will be viewed in the same light as other tumors whose molecular underpinnings have fueled the nascent age of precision medicine.

ACKNOWLEDGEMENT

The authors thank Michael Zhang for his invaluable help in preparation of this article.

REFERENCES

1. Ostrom QT, Gittleman H, Farah P, et al. CBTRUS statistical report: primary brain and central nervous system tumors diagnosed in the United States in 2006-2010. Neuro Oncol 2013;15(Suppl 2):ii1–56.
2. Herscovici Z, Rappaport Z, Sulkes J, et al. Natural history of conservatively treated meningiomas. Neurology 2004;63(6):1133–4.
3. Louis DN, Ohgaki H, Wiestler OD, et al. WHO classification of tumours of the central nervous system. 4th edition. Lyon (France): IARC Press; 2007.
4. Tanzler E, Morris CG, Kirwan JM, et al. Outcomes of WHO grade I meningiomas receiving definitive or postoperative radiotherapy. Int J Radiat Oncol Biol Phys 2011;79(2):508–13.
5. van Alkemade H, de Leau M, Dieleman EM, et al. Impaired survival and long-term neurological problems in benign meningioma. Neuro Oncol 2012; 14(5):658–66.
6. Rogers L, Barani I, Chamberlain M, et al. Meningiomas: knowledge base, treatment outcomes, and uncertainties. A RANO review. J Neurosurg 2015; 122(1):4–23.
7. Palma L, Celli P, Franco C, et al. Long-term prognosis for atypical and malignant meningiomas: a

study of 71 surgical cases. J Neurosurg 1997;86(5): 793–800.

8. Durand A, Labrousse F, Jouvet A, et al. WHO grade II and III meningiomas: a study of prognostic factors. J Neurooncol 2009;95(3):367–75.

9. Sun SQ, Kim AH, Cai C, et al. Management of atypical cranial meningiomas, part 1: predictors of recurrence and the role of adjuvant radiation after gross total resection. Neurosurgery 2014;75(4):347–54 [discussion: 354–5; quiz: 355].

10. Sun SQ, Cai C, Murphy RK, et al. Management of atypical cranial meningiomas, part 2: predictors of progression and the role of adjuvant radiation after subtotal resection. Neurosurgery 2014;75(4):356–63 [discussion: 363].

11. Palma L, Celli P, Franco C, et al. Long-term prognosis for atypical and malignant meningiomas: a study of 71 surgical cases. Neurosurg Focus 1997; 2(4):e3.

12. Witt H, Mack SC, Ryzhova M, et al. Delineation of two clinically and molecularly distinct subgroups of posterior fossa ependymoma. Cancer Cell 2011; 20(2):143–57.

13. Northcott PA, Korshunov A, Pfister SM, et al. The clinical implications of medulloblastoma subgroups. Nat Rev Neurol 2012;8(6):340–51.

14. Brennan CW, Verhaak RG, McKenna A, et al. The somatic genomic landscape of glioblastoma. Cell 2013;155(2):462–77.

15. Sosman JA, Kim KB, Schuchter L, et al. Survival in BRAF V600-mutant advanced melanoma treated with vemurafenib. N Engl J Med 2012;366(8):707–14.

16. Druker BJ, Talpaz M, Resta DJ, et al. Efficacy and safety of a specific inhibitor of the BCR-ABL tyrosine kinase in chronic myeloid leukemia. N Engl J Med 2001;344(14):1031–7.

17. Brastianos PK, Horowitz PM, Santagata S, et al. Genomic sequencing of meningiomas identifies oncogenic SMO and AKT1 mutations. Nat Genet 2013;45(3):285–9.

18. Clark VE, Erson-Omay EZ, Serin A, et al. Genomic analysis of non-NF2 meningiomas reveals mutations in TRAF7, KLF4, AKT1, and SMO. Science 2013; 339(6123):1077–80.

19. Bi WL, Abedalthagafi M, Horowitz P, et al. Genomic landscape of intracranial meningiomas. J Neurosurg 2016.

20. He S, Pham MH, Pease M, et al. A review of epigenetic and gene expression alterations associated with intracranial meningiomas. Neurosurg Focus 2013;35(6):E5.

21. Jones PA, Baylin SB. The fundamental role of epigenetic events in cancer. Nat Rev Genet 2002;3(6): 415–28.

22. Bello MJ, Aminoso C, Lopez-Marin I, et al. DNA methylation of multiple promoter-associated CpG islands in meningiomas: relationship with the allelic status at 1p and 22q. Acta Neuropathol 2004; 108(5):413–21.

23. Das PM, Singal R. DNA methylation and cancer. J Clin Oncol 2004;22(22):4632–42.

24. McDermott U, Downing JR, Stratton MR. Genomics and the continuum of cancer care. N Engl J Med 2011;364(4):340–50.

25. Cheishvili D, Boureau L, Szyf M. DNA demethylation and invasive cancer: implications for therapeutics. Br J Pharmacol 2015;172(11):2705–15.

26. Fontaine B, Rouleau GA, Seizinger BR, et al. Molecular genetics of neurofibromatosis 2 and related tumors (acoustic neuroma and meningioma). Ann N Y Acad Sci 1991;615:338–43.

27. Ruttledge MH, Sarrazin J, Rangaratnam S, et al. Evidence for the complete inactivation of the NF2 gene in the majority of sporadic meningiomas. Nat Genet 1994;6(2):180–4.

28. Perry A, Scheithauer BW, Stafford SL, et al. Malignancy" in meningiomas: a clinicopathologic study of 116 patients, with grading implications. Cancer 1999;85(9):2046–56.

29. Kalamarides M, Niwa-Kawakita M, Leblois H, et al. Nf2 gene inactivation in arachnoidal cells is rate-limiting for meningioma development in the mouse. Genes Dev 2002;16(9):1060–5.

30. Kalamarides M, Stemmer-Rachamimov AO, Niwa-Kawakita M, et al. Identification of a progenitor cell of origin capable of generating diverse meningioma histological subtypes. Oncogene 2011;30(20):2333–44.

31. Reuss DE, Piro RM, Jones DT, et al. Secretory meningiomas are defined by combined KLF4 K409Q and TRAF7 mutations. Acta Neuropathol 2013; 125(3):351–8.

32. Takahashi K, Tanabe K, Ohnuki M, et al. Induction of pluripotent stem cells from adult human fibroblasts by defined factors. Cell 2007;131(5): 861–72.

33. Sahm F, Bissel J, Koelsche C, et al. AKT1E17K mutations cluster with meningothelial and transitional meningiomas and can be detected by SFRP1 immunohistochemistry. Acta Neuropathol 2013;126(5): 757–62.

34. Bleeker FE, Felicioni L, Buttitta F, et al. AKT1(E17K) in human solid tumours. Oncogene 2008;27(42): 5648–50.

35. Reifenberger J, Wolter M, Weber RG, et al. Missense mutations in SMOH in sporadic basal cell carcinomas of the skin and primitive neuroectodermal tumors of the central nervous system. Cancer Res 1998;58(9):1798–803.

36. Jones DT, Jager N, Kool M, et al. Dissecting the genomic complexity underlying medulloblastoma. Nature 2012;488(7409):100–5.

37. Sekulic A, Migden MR, Oro AE, et al. Efficacy and safety of vismodegib in advanced basal-cell carcinoma. N Engl J Med 2012;366(23):2171–9.

38. Perry A, Louis DN, Scheithauer BW, et al. Meningiomas. In: Louis DN, Ohgaki H, Wiestler OD, et al, editors. WHO classification of tumours of the central nervous system. 4th edition. Lyon (France): IARC; 2007. p. 164–72.

39. Abedalthagafi MS, Merrill PH, Bi WL, et al. Angiomatous meningiomas have a distinct genetic profile with multiple chromosomal polysomies including polysomy of chromosome 5. Oncotarget 2014;5(21):10596–606.

40. Cai DX, Banerjee R, Scheithauer BW, et al. Chromosome 1p and 14q FISH analysis in clinicopathologic subsets of meningioma: diagnostic and prognostic implications. J Neuropathol Exp Neurol 2001;60(6): 628–36.

41. Buschges R, Ichimura K, Weber RG, et al. Allelic gain and amplification on the long arm of chromosome 17 in anaplastic meningiomas. Brain Pathol 2002;12(2):145–53.

42. Lomas J, Aminoso C, Gonzalez-Gomez P, et al. Methylation status of TP73 in meningiomas. Cancer Genet Cytogenet 2004;148(2):148–51.

43. Lusis EA, Watson MA, Chicoine MR, et al. Integrative genomic analysis identifies NDRG2 as a candidate tumor suppressor gene frequently inactivated in clinically aggressive meningioma. Cancer Res 2005;65(16):7121–6.

44. Liu Y, Pang JC, Dong S, et al. Aberrant CpG island hypermethylation profile is associated with atypical and anaplastic meningiomas. Hum Pathol 2005; 36(4):416–25.

45. Carling T, Kim KC, Yang XH, et al. A histone methyltransferase is required for maximal response to female sex hormones. Mol Cell Biol 2004;24(16):7032–42.

46. Chadwick RB, Jiang GL, Bennington GA, et al. Candidate tumor suppressor RIZ is frequently involved in colorectal carcinogenesis. Proc Natl Acad Sci U S A 2000;97(6):2662–7.

47. He L, Yu JX, Liu L, et al. RIZ1, but not the alternative RIZ2 product of the same gene, is underexpressed in breast cancer, and forced RIZ1 expression causes G2-M cell cycle arrest and/or apoptosis. Cancer Res 1998;58(19):4238–44.

48. Jiang G, Liu L, Buyse IM, et al. Decreased RIZ1 expression but not RIZ2 in hepatoma and suppression of hepatoma tumorigenicity by RIZ1. Int J Cancer 1999;83(4):541–6.

49. Liu ZY, Wang JY, Liu HH, et al. Retinoblastoma protein-interacting zinc-finger gene 1 (RIZ1) dysregulation in human malignant meningiomas. Oncogene 2013;32(10):1216–22.

50. Ding MH, Wang Z, Jiang L, et al. The transducible TAT-RIZ1-PR protein exerts histone methyltransferase activity and tumor-suppressive functions in human malignant meningiomas. Biomaterials 2015;56:165–78.

51. Rauch T, Wang Z, Zhang X, et al. Homeobox gene methylation in lung cancer studied by genome-wide analysis with a microarray-based methylated CpG island recovery assay. Proc Natl Acad Sci U S A 2007;104(13):5527–32.

52. Wu Q, Lothe RA, Ahlquist T, et al. DNA methylation profiling of ovarian carcinomas and their in vitro models identifies HOXA9, HOXB5, SCGB3A1, and CRABP1 as novel targets. Mol Cancer 2007;6:45.

53. Kishida Y, Natsume A, Kondo Y, et al. Epigenetic subclassification of meningiomas based on genome-wide DNA methylation analyses. Carcinogenesis 2012;33(2):436–41.

54. Ando H, Natsume A, Senga T, et al. Peptide-based inhibition of the HOXA9/PBX interaction retards the growth of human meningioma. Cancer Chemother Pharmacol 2014;73(1):53–60.

55. Jun P, Hong C, Lal A, et al. Epigenetic silencing of the kinase tumor suppressor WNK2 is tumor-type and tumor-grade specific. Neuro Oncol 2009;11(4): 414–22.

56. Moniz S, Verissimo F, Matos P, et al. Protein kinase WNK2 inhibits cell proliferation by negatively modulating the activation of MEK1/ERK1/2. Oncogene 2007;26(41):6071–81.

57. Gao F, Shi L, Russin J, et al. DNA methylation in the malignant transformation of meningiomas. PLoS One 2013;8(1):e54114.

58. Smith MJ, O'Sullivan J, Bhaskar SS, et al. Loss-of-function mutations in SMARCE1 cause an inherited disorder of multiple spinal meningiomas. Nat Genet 2013;45(3):295–8.

59. Smith MJ, Wallace AJ, Bennett C, et al. Germline SMARCE1 mutations predispose to both spinal and cranial clear cell meningiomas. J Pathol 2014; 234(4):436–40.

60. Kros J, de Greve K, van Tilborg A, et al. NF2 status of meningiomas is associated with tumour localization and histology. J Pathol 2001;194(3):367–72.

61. Di Vinci A, Brigati C, Casciano I, et al. HOXA7, 9, and 10 are methylation targets associated with aggressive behavior in meningiomas. Transl Res 2012;160(5):355–62.

62. Barski D, Wolter M, Reifenberger G, et al. Hypermethylation and transcriptional downregulation of the TIMP3 gene is associated with allelic loss on 22q12.3 and malignancy in meningiomas. Brain Pathol 2010;20(3):623–31.

63. Nakane Y, Natsume A, Wakabayashi T, et al. Malignant transformation-related genes in meningiomas: allelic loss on 1p36 and methylation status of p73 and RASSF1A. J Neurosurg 2007;107(2): 398–404.

64. Lee JY, Finkelstein S, Hamilton RL, et al. Loss of heterozygosity analysis of benign, atypical, and anaplastic meningiomas. Neurosurgery 2004;55(5): 1163–73.

65. Lamszus K, Kluwe L, Matschke J, et al. Allelic losses at 1p, 9q, 10q, 14q, and 22q in the progression of aggressive meningiomas and undifferentiated

meningeal sarcomas. Cancer Genet Cytogenet 1999;110(2):103–10.

66. Aizer AA, Abedalthagafi M, Bi WL, et al. A prognostic cytogenetic scoring system to guide the adjuvant management of patients with atypical meningioma. Neuro Oncol 2016;18(2):269–74.

67. Langford LA, Piatyszek MA, Xu R, et al. Telomerase activity in ordinary meningiomas predicts poor outcome. Hum Pathol 1997;28(4):416–20.

68. Sawyer JR, Husain M, Pravdenkova S, et al. A role for telomeric and centromeric instability in the progression of chromosome aberrations in meningioma patients. Cancer 2000;88(2):440–53.

69. Chen HJ, Liang CL, Lu K, et al. Implication of telomerase activity and alternations of telomere length in the histologic characteristics of intracranial meningiomas. Cancer 2000;89(10):2092–8.

70. Simon M, Park TW, Leuenroth S, et al. Telomerase activity and expression of the telomerase catalytic subunit, hTERT, in meningioma progression. J Neurosurg 2000;92(5):832–40.

71. Leuraud P, Dezamis E, Aguirre-Cruz L, et al. Prognostic value of allelic losses and telomerase activity in meningiomas. J Neurosurg 2004;100(2):303–9.

72. Goutagny S, Nault JC, Mallet M, et al. High incidence of activating TERT promoter mutations in meningiomas undergoing malignant progression. Brain Pathol 2014;24(2):184–9.

73. Zhi F, Zhou G, Wang S, et al. A microRNA expression signature predicts meningioma recurrence. Int J Cancer 2013;132(1):128–36.

74. Melino G, De Laurenzi V, Vousden KH. p73: Friend or foe in tumorigenesis. Nat Rev Cancer 2002;2(8):605–15.

75. Zhang X, Gejman R, Mahta A, et al. Maternally expressed gene 3, an imprinted noncoding RNA gene, is associated with meningioma pathogenesis and progression. Cancer Res 2010;70(6):2350–8.

76. Lu Z, Lam KS, Wang N, et al. LMO4 can interact with Smad proteins and modulate transforming growth factor-beta signaling in epithelial cells. Oncogene 2006;25(20):2920–30.

77. Cuevas IC, Slocum AL, Jun P, et al. Meningioma transcript profiles reveal deregulated Notch signaling pathway. Cancer Res 2005;65(12):5070–5.

78. Keller A, Ludwig N, Backes C, et al. Genome wide expression profiling identifies specific deregulated pathways in meningioma. Int J Cancer 2009;124(2):346–51.

79. Larijani L, Madjd Z, Samadikuchaksaraei A, et al. Methylation of O6-methyl guanine methyltransferase gene promoter in meningiomas–comparison between tumor grades I, II, and III. Asian Pac J Cancer Prev 2014;15(1):33–8.

80. Saydam O, Shen Y, Wurdinger T, et al. Downregulated microRNA-200a in meningiomas promotes tumor growth by reducing E-cadherin and activating the Wnt/beta-catenin signaling pathway. Mol Cell Biol 2009;29(21):5923–40.

81. Panetti TS, Chen H, Misenheimer TM, et al. Endothelial cell mitogenesis induced by LPA: inhibition by thrombospondin-1 and thrombospondin-2. J Lab Clin Med 1997;129(2):208–16.

82. Ando H, Natsume A, Iwami K, et al. A hypoxia-inducible factor (HIF)-3alpha splicing variant, HIF-3alpha4 impairs angiogenesis in hypervascular malignant meningiomas with epigenetically silenced HIF-3alpha4. Biochem Biophys Res Commun 2013;433(1):139–44.

83. Vengoechea J, Sloan AE, Chen Y, et al. Methylation markers of malignant potential in meningiomas. J Neurosurg 2013;119(4):899–906.

84. Kandenwein JA, Park-Simon TW, Schramm J, et al. uPA/PAI-1 expression and uPA promoter methylation in meningiomas. J Neurooncol 2011;103(3):533–9.

85. Velpula KK, Gogineni VR, Nalla AK, et al. Radiation-induced hypomethylation triggers urokinase plasminogen activator transcription in meningioma cells. Neoplasia 2013;15(2):192–203.

86. Nordqvist AC, Peyrard M, Pettersson H, et al. A high ratio of insulin-like growth factor II/insulin-like growth factor binding protein 2 messenger RNA as a marker for anaplasia in meningiomas. Cancer Res 1997;57(13):2611–4.

87. Wrobel G, Roerig P, Kokocinski F, et al. Microarray-based gene expression profiling of benign, atypical and anaplastic meningiomas identifies novel genes associated with meningioma progression. Int J Cancer 2005;114(2):249–56.

88. Ioannidis P, Mahaira LG, Perez SA, et al. CRD-BP/IMP1 expression characterizes cord blood CD34+ stem cells and affects c-myc and IGF-II expression in MCF-7 cancer cells. J Biol Chem 2005;280(20):20086–93.

89. Kliese N, Gobrecht P, Pachow D, et al. miRNA-145 is downregulated in atypical and anaplastic meningiomas and negatively regulates motility and proliferation of meningioma cells. Oncogene 2013;32(39):4712–20.

90. Perez-Magan E, Campos-Martin Y, Mur P, et al. Genetic alterations associated with progression and recurrence in meningiomas. J Neuropathol Exp Neurol 2012;71(10):882–93.

91. Perez-Magan E, Rodriguez de Lope A, Ribalta T, et al. Differential expression profiling analyses identifies downregulation of 1p, 6q, and 14q genes and overexpression of 6p histone cluster 1 genes as markers of recurrence in meningiomas. Neuro Oncol 2010;12(12):1278–90.

92. Linsler S, Kraemer D, Driess C, et al. Molecular biological determinations of meningioma progression and recurrence. PLoS One 2014;9(4):e94987.

Secretory Meningiomas
Characteristic Features and Clinical Management of a Unique Subgroup

Malte Mohme, MD[a], Pedram Emami, MD[a],
Jakob Matschke, MD[b], Jan Regelsberger, MD[a],
Manfred Westphal, MD[a], Sven Oliver Eicker, MD[a],*

KEYWORDS

• Meningioma • Secretory • Edema • Management

KEY POINTS

• Secretory meningiomas (SM) frequently present with extensive and disproportional peritumoral edema, which can complicate the clinical course and have a direct impact on prognosis and outcome.
• SM represent a benign histologic subgroup defined by a glandular transformation and the appearance of periodic-acidic Schiff–positive pseudopsammomas.
• This subgroup is characterized by an exclusive mutation in the KLF4 gene (K409Q) and a presumably interdependent mutation in the *TRAF7* gene.

INTRODUCTION

Secretory meningiomas (SM) represent a rare variant of the most common benign intracranial brain tumor. Defined by the histologic appearance of eosinophilic glandular formations and periodic-acidic Schiff (PAS)-positive pseudopsammoma bodies, SM are characterized by unique molecular alterations, a disproportional occurrence of reactive peritumoral brain edema (PTBE), and a clinical course that demands for increased awareness for perioperative complications. The frequent presence of extensive peritumoral edema has become a hallmark of SM and can be associated with life-threatening complications.[1] Although the exact pathophysiology of edema formation in SM is still unknown, the study of larger case series and the recent discovery of exclusive molecular alteration have helped to gain new insights into the unique clinical presentation of this distinct meningioma subgroup.

CLINICAL PRESENTATION AND IMAGING

SM are predominantly seen in female patients in the fifth decade. Interestingly, with a female-to-male ratio of 3:1 up to 11:1,[1–6] the prevalence of SM in women significantly exceeds the ratio of 2:1 described for meningiomas in general.[7] Similar to other benign meningioma subtypes, SM exhibit slow extra-axial growth. Usually this slow growth pattern results in the compression of adjacent structures, like cranial nerves or brain parenchyma, which consecutively leads to the clinical presentation depending on the location of the tumor. Besides unspecific headache, symptoms of cranial nerve compression, vertigo, focal seizures, diplopia, or other focal neurologic deficits are observed. Extremely rarely, SM can present with unusual symptoms like a transformed migraine or otitis media-like syndrome.[8,9] The pronounced edema leads to a shorter time to diagnosis and an increased likelihood of symptoms,

The authors have no financial or personal interest in the materials and devices described.
[a] Department of Neurosurgery, University Medical Center Hamburg Eppendorf, Martinistr. 52, Hamburg 20246, Germany; [b] Department of Neuropathology, University Medical Center Hamburg Eppendorf, Martinistr. 52, Hamburg 20246, Germany
* Corresponding author.
E-mail address: s.eicker@uke.de

Neurosurg Clin N Am 27 (2016) 181–187
http://dx.doi.org/10.1016/j.nec.2015.11.001

neurosurgery.theclinics.com

which in turn is associated with higher rate of post-surgical complications (13.6% in asymptomatic vs 21.7% in symptomatic patients), as demonstrated by a study from Zeng and colleagues.[10,11]

On MRI, SM present as an extra-axial mass of dural origin, which appears isointense or hypointense in T1-, and hyperintense or isointense on T2-weighted images, with homogenous enhancement after application of contrasting agents such as gadolinium (**Fig. 1**).[12] SM can cause hyperostosis of the adjacent bone (13%), are frequently located at the skull base, and had intratumoral calcifications in 8.3% of cases.[3] Although other benign meningioma subgroups usually provoke reactive changes in a moderate extent or no changes in the adjacent brain parenchyma, SM are different in this regard. Extensive or even severe hemispheric PTBE was observed in 13% to 64% of all patients (**Fig. 2, Table 1**).[1–5] Exceeding the size of its originating tumor, this edema frequently resulted in a significant midline shift of greater than 10 mm and can be made responsible for an increased prevalence of perioperative and intraoperative complications, including progressive neurologic symptoms or loss of consciousness during the postoperative period.[1,3] Interestingly, more severe PTBE was observed in SM presenting with irregular margins, absence of peritumoral rim, and non-skull-base location.[3]

HISTOPATHOLOGY AND GENETICS

Meningiomas are slow-growing extra-axial tumors of the central nervous system, originating from arachnoidal cap cells. Among the 15 different meningioma variants, SM represent a benign subgroup with a prevalence of 1.1% to 4.4% and a unique epithelial and secretory transformation.[1,6,7,13–15] Only in extremely rare cases, an anaplastic variant or a progression to a higher grade (World Health Organization [WHO] II) has been documented.[16,17]

First described by Harvey Cushing and Louise Eisenhardt,[18] SM are defined by glandlike eosinophilic hyaline inclusions within intracytoplasmic lumina, which are lined by microvilli, also called pseudopsammomas.[2] These PAS-positive globules are pathognomonic for the SM subtype and show strong correlation to the characteristic PTBE formation.[1,2] Labeling with carcinoembryonic antigen (CEA) and broad-spectrum cytokeratin (CK) shows characteristic focal CEA and CK positivity surrounding the pseudopsammomas (**Fig. 3**). The secretory characteristics do not correlate to MIB-1 proliferation index.[1] Additional studies further report positivity for the epithelial

membrane antigen (EMA), CK7, CK8, as well as certain mucin epitopes, including sialyl-Tn, Tn, CA19.9, CA125, while staining for CK20, CD15, and BerEP4 are negative.[19,20] Because the histologic glandular formation of SM can impose a histopathological characteristic similar to metastatic adenocarcinoma, the differential expression of CK7 and CK20 can aid in the differential diagnosis (CK7+/CK20− for SM, CK7−/CK20+ for adenocarcinoma).[20]

SM exhibit high rates of progesterone and estrogen receptor positivity (33%–100%),[1,4,15] which is in concordance with the female preponderance in the prevalence rate. First, histologic evidence for the unique pathophysiology of SM was described by Paek and colleagues,[21] who demonstrated a link between vascular endothelial growth factor (VEGF) and matrix metalloproteinase -9 expression to the peritumoral edema. Furthermore, additional evidence was found in an increased frequency of CD117-positive mast cells as well as the pronounced pericytic proliferation patterns within the vessel walls (83%–92% of SM) compared with meningotheliomatous meningiomas.[4,5]

Complementing histopathological investigations in unraveling the pathogenesis of SM, a recently published whole-exome sequencing analysis of 16 SM for the first time described that SM are defined by the combination of Kruppel-like factor-4 (*KLF4*) and *Tumor necrosis factor Receptor-Associated Factor 7* (*TRAF7*) mutations.[22] Again emphasizing the unique role of the secretory subgroup, identical heterozygous *KLF4* mutations (K409Q in exon 4 on chromosome 9q) were found in 100% of SM tumors, while were absent in other meningioma subgroups or other types of intracranial tumors. *KLF4* is supposed to play a role in oncogenic activation, tumor suppression, and stem-cell maintenance.[22] The second mutation was described in the *TRAF7* gene. Although *KLF4* was exclusive to SM, *TRAF7* mutations could be detected in 93% of SM and 8% of non-SM (meningotheliomatous and atypical). Influencing signal transduction, *TRAF7* inhibits NF-κB activation and serves as an agonist for the JNK-AP1 pathway. Interestingly, supporting an *NF2*-independent pathogenesis in SM,[23] *NF2* mutations could only be detected in meningiomas with no *KLF4* or *TRAF7* mutations.[22,24] The tight linkage of these 2 mutations highlights the interplay of interdependent mutational incidents in SM cancerogenesis.[22] Furthermore, the discovery of the exclusiveness of the *KLF4* K409Q mutations supports the notion to consider SM as a separate meningioma entity.

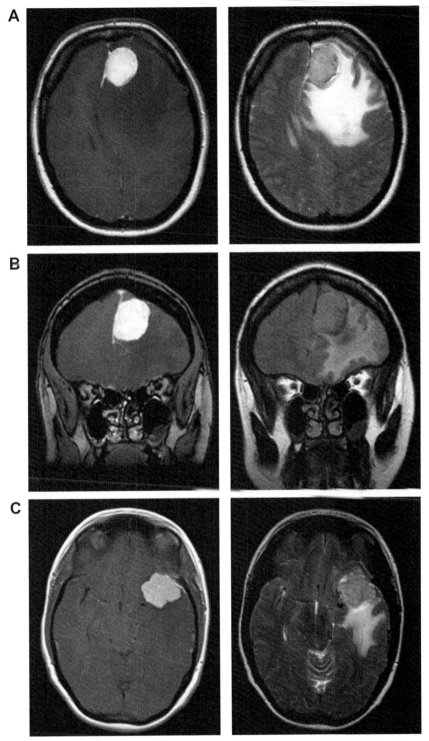

Fig. 1. MRI of 2 representative secretory meningioma patients with extensive peritumoral white matter edema and midline shift (*A* and *B*: case 1; *C*: case 2) depicted in contrast-enhanced T1- (*left*) and T2-weighted (*right*) images. (*Courtesy of* Dr E. Goebell and Dr J. Fiehler, Department of Neuroradiology, University Medical Center Hamburg–Eppendorf, Hamburg, Germany.)

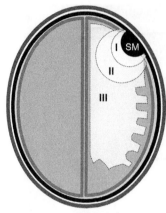

Fig. 2. Schematic drawing of perifocal edema extension around the tumor (SM) and its classification by using the scoring system. (*From* Regelsberger J, Hagel C, Emami P, et al. Secretory meningiomas: a benign subgroup causing life-threatening complications. Neuro Oncol 2009;11(6):819–24.)

CLINICAL MANAGEMENT AND COMPLICATIONS

Although up to 99% of all meningiomas are slow-growing WHO I and II neoplasms, this tumor can produce significant morbidity.[25] As mentioned above, clinical symptoms usually present due to the mass effect and the compression of adjacent structures. Furthermore, 60% of all meningiomas are associated with PTBE.[26] Ample studies have shown that this PTBE has significant impact on clinical course and prognosis of meningiomas, and therefore, has to be treated with additional awareness, especially in this unique entity of meningioma.

A variety of factors causing PTBE have been proposed, including tumor size, location, venous compression, vascularity, secretory activity, immune cell infiltration, and hormone receptor composition.[27–29] Because the edema is located within white matter and the tumor is separated by the arachnoid membrane, which is impermeable to water,[30] the pia mater, which is impermeable to edema-causing macromolecules,[31] and by the densely cellular cerebral cortex, a further correlation between PTBE and cortical invasion, as well as disruption of the tumor-brain barrier, has been hypothesized.[25,26,29] Another theory postulates the involvement of cerebral pial vessel recruitment as a critical factor for edema formation.[32] Together with the fact that PTBE is associated with irregular tumor margins,[3,29] these observations implicate the loss of a clear anatomic dissection plane and a higher prevalence of surgical complications.[33] Furthermore, the pre-existing edema demands for an adjustment in the surgical approach. For example, large craniotomies are undesirably and even more are large dural openings because this allows the edematous brain to herniate out of the exposure, resulting in further compressive ischemia at the margins of the dural opening and the beginning of a viscous cycle. Therefore, in the case of a convexity meningioma, careful planning of the extent of the dural opening by transdural ultrasound is recommended. The dural opening should then be slightly inside the margins of the tumor, followed by debulking to gain space for resection of the margins. Because PTBE was even more pronounced in SM of the convexity, this recommendation also applies for non-cranial-base SM.[1,3,29] Edema surrounding tumors in eloquent areas are further associated with increased risk for postoperative neurologic deficits.[34] In addition, PTBE in meningiomas was also associated with increased rate of blood supply from the internal carotid artery, pial vessel formation, and a higher risk to require blood transfusions.[29,33] The surgeon should take these facts into consideration, especially when PTBE is present and no clear arachnoid plane can be demonstrated on preoperative MRI scans. Unfortunately, at this point, there are no data about the rate of recurrence or the overall prognosis specific for this subgroup. Retrospective analysis of SM operated at the authors' institution showed that 23.7% (9/38) of cases needed a second surgical intervention, which is greater than the reported recurrence rate of 7% to 20% in WHO I meningioma.[7]

Taken together, preoperative attenuation of PTBE is desirable to decrease intraoperative and postoperative complications.[1,25] Because of their long-proven efficacy in reducing vasogenic edema in malignant brain tumors, the most widely used

Table 1
Edema scores for secretory meningiomas

Edema Score[1]:	
I	Equal or smaller than tumor size
II	Bigger than tumor size
III	Extensive/hemispheric edema

Edema Score[14]:	
Small	Smaller than tumor size
Moderate	Equal to tumor size
Severe	Bigger than tumor size

Data from Regelsberger J, Hagel C, Emami P, et al. Secretory meningiomas: a benign subgroup causing life-threatening complications. Neuro Oncol 2009; 11(6):819–24; and Buhl R, Hugo HH, Mehdorn HM. Brain oedema in secretory meningiomas. J Clin Neurosci 2001;8(Suppl 1):19–21.

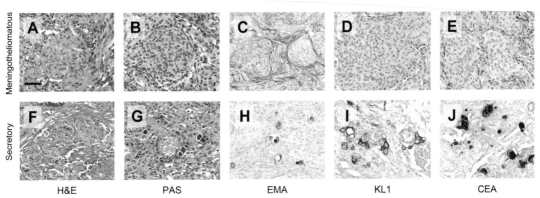

Fig. 3. Comparison of histologic appearance of secretory (*F–J*) and meningotheliomatous (*A–E*) meningiomas with hematoxylin & eosin (H&E), PAS, EMA, KL1, and CEA stainings of formalin-fixed paraffin-embedded tumor tissue. Bar indicates 50 μm.

antiedematous agents in clinical practice are corticosteroids. However, the efficacy of cortico steroids in PTBE of meningioma is controversial.[25,35,36] Usually steroids result in progressive decrease of PTBE by an average of 50% after 1 week of treatment.[37] Although comparable to malignant tumors, the edemagenesis in meningioma is described to be vasogenic, the sensitivity to corticosteroids is reduced.[36,37] As VEGF-A is suspected to play a pathophysiological role in PTBE in meningioma, anti-angiogenic drugs have been implicated in the perioperative treatment.[25,38,39] Unfortunately, because of the tremendous costs and their contraindication in surgical settings, antiangiogenic drugs targeting VEGF-A will not move into clinical practice In the near future and alternative antiedema compounds, like cyclo-oxygenase-2 as well as boswellic acids, will have to pass clinical testing for this application.[25,40] Therefore, currently no recommendations regarding the use of systemic therapy can be made for this histologic subtype. In addition, because so far only scarce data are available on the expression of hormonal receptors in SM, current guidelines regarding discontinuation of estrogen and progesterone medications can be adapted from the common meningotheliomatous histologic subtype.

The higher risk of postoperative complications in SM includes intracranial hematoma, raised intracranial pressure postoperatively despite surgical tumor removal likely to be seen in an increased vulnerability of the edematous brain even to careful surgical manipulation; this results in prolonged intensive care unit and hospital stay as well as a worse outcome.[1,3,29,33,41] Notably, in 40% of SM patients with extensive PTBE, edema formation continued or increased after surgical intervention, and 34% of patients experienced progressive neurologic symptoms or even loss of consciousness postoperatively.[1] To confirm suspected diagnosis of SM, intraoperative frozen sections with a focused PAS staining are helpful to prepare for optimal postsurgical care to lower the threshold for antiedematous therapy or postoperative imaging.[1]

SUMMARY

Because of their defined glandular transformation and the pathognomonic appearance of PAS-positive pseudopsammomas, as well as their exclusive mutations in the *KLF4* and *TRAF7* genes, SM represent a rare, but very unique subgroup of meningiomas. Furthermore, the frequently observed extensive peritumoral edema can complicate the clinical and surgical management In order to anticipate the impact of perifocal edema on symptoms, postoperative complications, and prognostic outcome caused by SM, neurosurgeons should be aware of the characteristic features of this benign subgroup.

REFERENCES

1. Regelsberger J, Hagel C, Emami P, et al. Secretory meningiomas: a benign subgroup causing life-threatening complications. Neuro Oncol 2009; 11(6):819–24.
2. Probst-Cousin S, Villagran-Lillo R, Lahl R, et al. Secretory meningioma: clinical, histologic, and immunohistochemical findings in 31 cases. Cancer 1997;79(10):2003–15.
3. Wang DJ, Xie Q, Gong Y, et al. Secretory meningiomas: clinical, radiological and pathological findings in 70 consecutive cases at one institution. Int J Clin Exp Pathol 2013;6(3):358–74.
4. Colakoğlu N, Demirtaş E, Oktar N, et al. Secretory meningiomas. J Neurooncol 2003;62(3):233–41.

5. Tirakotai W, Mennel HD, Celik I, et al. Secretory meningioma: immunohistochemical findings and evaluation of mast cell infiltration. Neurosurg Rev 2006;29(1):41–8.

6. Kamp MA, Beseoglu K, Eicker S, et al. Secretory meningiomas: systematic analysis of epidemiological, clinical, and radiological features. Acta Neurochir (Wien) 2011;153(3):457–65.

7. Lamszus K. Meningioma pathology, genetics, and biology. J Neuropathol Exp Neurol 2004;63(4):275–86.

8. Marcelissen TAT, De Bondt RBJ, Lammens M, et al. Primary temporal bone secretory meningioma presenting as chronic otitis media. Eur Arch Otorhinolaryngol 2008;265(7):843–6.

9. Evans RW, Timm JS, Baskin DS. A left frontal secretory meningioma can mimic transformed migraine with and without aura. Headache 2015;55(6):849–52.

10. Trittmacher S, Traupe H, Schmid A, et al. Pre- and postoperative changes in brain tissue surrounding a meningioma. Neurosurgery 1988;22(5):882–5.

11. Zeng L, Wang L, Ye F, et al. Clinical characteristics of patients with asymptomatic intracranial meningiomas and results of their surgical management. Neurosurg Rev 2015;38(3):481–8.

12. Nishio S, Morioka T, Suzuki S, et al. Secretory meningioma: clinicopathologic features of eight cases. J Clin Neurosci 2001;8(4):335–9.

13. Louis DN, Ohgaki H, Wiestler OD, et al. The 2007 WHO classification of tumours of the central nervous system. Acta Neuropathol 2007;114(2):97–109.

14. Buhl R, Hugo HH, Mehdorn HM. Brain oedema in secretory meningiomas. J Clin Neurosci 2001;8(Suppl 1):19–21.

15. Buhl R, Hugo HH, Mihajlovic Z, et al. Secretory meningiomas: clinical and immunohistochemical observations. Neurosurgery 2001;48(2):297–302.

16. Ferchichi L, Bellil S, Ben HK, et al. Anaplastic secretory meningioma: a case report. Pathologica 2006;98(2):153–5.

17. Shivane AG, Chakrabarty A, Baborie A, et al. A rare case of recurrent secretory meningioma with malignant transformation. Br J Neurosurg 2006;20:250–3.

18. Cushing H, Eisenhardt L. Meningiomas. Their classification, regional behaviour, life history, and surgical end results. Br J Surg 1939;26(104):957.

19. Taraszewska A, Matyja E. Secretory meningiomas: immunohistochemical pattern of lectin and ultrastructure of pseudopsammoma bodies. Folia Neuropathol 2014;52(2):141–50.

20. Assi A, Declich P, Iacobellis M, et al. Secretory meningioma, a rare meningioma subtype with characteristic glandular differentation: an histological and immunohistochemical study of 9 cases. Adv Clin Path 1999;3(3):47–53.

21. Paek SH, Kim CY, Kim YY, et al. Correlation of clinical and biological parameters with peritumoral edema in meningioma. J Neurooncol 2002;60(3):235–45.

22. Reuss DE, Piro RM, Jones DT, et al. Secretory meningiomas are defined by combined KLF4 K409Q and TRAF7 mutations. Acta Neuropathol 2013;125(3):351–8.

23. Hartmann C, Sieberns J, Gehlhaar C, et al. NF2 mutations in secretory and other rare variants of meningiomas. Brain Pathol 2006;16(1):15–9.

24. Buccoliero AM, Gheri CF, Castiglione F, et al. Merlin expression in secretory meningiomas: evidence of an NF2-independent pathogenesis? Immunohistochemical study. Appl Immunohistochem Mol Morphol 2007;15:353–7.

25. Hou J, Kshettry VR, Selman WR, et al. Peritumoral brain edema in intracranial meningiomas: the emergence of vascular endothelial growth factor-directed therapy. Neurosurg Focus 2013;35(6):E2.

26. Simis A, Pires de Aguiar PH, Leite CC, et al. Peritumoral brain edema in benign meningiomas: correlation with clinical, radiologic, and surgical factors and possible role on recurrence. Surg Neurol 2008;70(5):471–7.

27. Yoshioka H, Hama S, Taniguchi E, et al. Peritumoral brain edema associated with meningioma: influence of vascular endothelial growth factor expression and vascular blood supply. Cancer 1999;85(4):936–44.

28. Tanaka M, Imhof HG, Schucknecht B, et al. Correlation between the efferent venous drainage of the tumor and peritumoral edema in intracranial meningiomas: superselective angiographic analysis of 25 cases. J Neurosurg 2006;104(3):382–8.

29. Vignes JR, Sesay M, Rezajooi K, et al. Peritumoral edema and prognosis in intracranial meningioma surgery. J Clin Neurosci 2008;15(7):764–8.

30. Ildan F, Tuna M, Göçer AP, et al. Correlation of the relationships of brain-tumor interfaces, magnetic resonance imaging, and angiographic findings to predict cleavage of meningiomas. J Neurosurg 1999;91(3):384–90.

31. Gilbert JJ, Paulseth JE, Coates RK, et al. Cerebral edema associated with meningiomas. Neurosurgery 1983;12(6):599–605.

32. Bitzer M, Wöckel L, Luft AR, et al. The importance of pial blood supply to the development of peritumoral brain edema in meningiomas. J Neurosurg 1997;87(3):368–73.

33. Alaywan M, Sindou M. Prognostic factors in the surgery for intracranial meningioma. Role of the tumoral size and arterial vascularization originating from the pia mater. Study of 150 cases. Neurochirurgie 1993;39(6):337–47.

34. Sindou MP, Alaywan M. Most intracranial meningiomas are not cleavable tumors: anatomic-surgical evidence and angiographic predictibility. Neurosurgery 1998;42(3):476–80.

35. Skjoeth J, Bjerre PK. Effect of glucocorticoids on ICP in patients with a cerebral tumour. Acta Neurol Scand 1997;96(3):167–70.

36. Andersen C, Astrup J, Gyldensted C. Quantitative MR analysis of glucocorticoid effects on peritumoral edema associated with intracranial meningiomas and metastases. J Comput Assist Tomogr 1994; 18(4):509–18.

37. Jarden JO, Dhawan V, Moeller JR, et al. The time course of steroid action on blood-to-brain and blood-to-tumor transport of 82Rb: a positron emission tomographic study. Ann Neurol 1989;25(3): 239–45.

38. Markovic M, Antunovic V, Milenkovic S, et al. Prognostic value of peritumoral edema and angiogenesis in intracranial meningioma surgery. J BUON 2013; 18(2):430–6.

39. Lamszus K, Lengler U, Schmidt NO, et al. Vascular endothelial growth factor, hepatocyte growth factor/scatter factor, basic fibroblast growth factor, and placenta growth factor in human meningiomas and their relation to angiogenesis and malignancy. Neurosurgery 2000;46(4):938–47 [discussion: 947–8].

40. Wick W, Küker W. Brain edema in neurooncology: radiological assessment and management. Onkologie 2004;27:261–6.

41. Ouyang T, Zhang N, Wang L, et al. Sphenoid wing meningiomas: surgical strategies and evaluation of prognostic factors influencing clinical outcomes. Clin Neurol Neurosurg 2015;134:85–90.

Primary Intraosseous Meningioma

Thomas C. Chen, MD, PhD

KEYWORDS

- Intraosseous meningioma • Extradural meningioma • Surgical resection • Arachnoid cells

KEY POINTS

- Intraosseous meningiomas are rare lesions that originate in the skull and represent the most common type of extradural meningioma; the lesions are often asymptomatic but can cause proptosis and neurologic symptoms depending on their size and location.
- Intraosseous meningiomas likely originate from entrapment of arachnoid cells within the bone.
- The treatment of choice is surgical resection, which is potentially curative.
- Using 3-D neuronavigation and operative planning, tumor resection and cranioplasty may be performed simultaneously.
- Tumors that cannot be completely resected may require consideration for adjuvant therapy; this may include radiation therapy, chemotherapy, and/or etidronate.
- Further work is required to elucidate any optimal adjuvant therapy regimens.

INCIDENCE

A majority of meningiomas are considered primary intradural meningiomas (PIMs) and are located in the subdural space. By contrast, extradural meningiomas arise in locations other than the dura, such as the skin, nasopharynx, and neck.[1,2] Extradural meningiomas comprise 1% to 2% of all meningiomas.[3] *Primary intraosseous meningioma* is a term used to describe a subset of extradural meningiomas that arise in the skull. They represent approximately two-thirds of all extradural meningiomas.[2] A review of the literature reveals approximately 200 reported cases of intraosseous meningioma. This number has increased dramatically over the past decade. An article in 1995 presented the 36th case to the literature, whereas a publication 5 years later reviewed 168 cases of calvarial meningioma. Rather than a higher incidence, this increase in published cases likely represents a combination of improved histopathologic capabilities, such as immunostaining, as well as increased penetrance of radiographic techniques, such as MRI.

This article reviews the radiographic and clinical findings of patients with primary intraosseous meningiomas. Differential diagnosis, nomenclature, and treatment options are also discussed. The literature regarding these tumors is reviewed.

ETIOLOGY

Different theories exist regarding the origin of intraosseous meningiomas. Three main theories exist. First, arachnoidal cells on blood vessels or nerves traversing the skull may explain the origin of some intraosseous meningiomas.[4] Cellular dedifferentiation within the skull could also possibly explain the formation of an intraosseous meningioma.[5] Some investigators observed a possible trend for intraosseous meningiomas found predominantly near previous fracture sites or at suture lines, most commonly the coronal or pterion sutures.[6,7] Intraosseous meningiomas are thought to arise from arachnoidal cap cells caught in-between cranial sutures during birth, with subsequent modeling of the infant skull leading to intraosseous meningomas. The bony orbit and frontoparietal skull are the most common locations; however, they can theoretically arise from any location where there is cranial suture closure. Extradural

Neurosurgery and Pathology, University of Southern California, 1200, N state st suite 3300, Los Angeles, CA 90033, USA
E-mail address: tchen@med.usc.edu

Neurosurg Clin N Am 27 (2016) 189–193
http://dx.doi.org/10.1016/j.nec.2015.11.011

tumors may arise from cells that become misplaced after differentiation into meningocytes or arachnoid cap cells. Intraosseous meningiomas are thought to originate from arachnoid cap cells trapped in the cranial sutures, which may occur during molding of the cranium at birth.[8–10] Another theory involves meningothelial cells becoming trapped within skull fractures or sutures as a result of trauma.[11,12] Recently published case series, however, do not usually support these 2 theories.[6] A recent report published in 2000 reviewed 168 cases of calvarial meningiomas reported in the literature. Only 14 of these cases (8%) were associated with a cranial suture.[2] A separate report reviewed 36 cases in the literature and found that only 5 (14%) were associated with a history of head trauma in the region of the tumor.[13] Lastly, the concept of ectopic arachnoid cap cells giving rise to intraosseous meningiomas should be considered. In general, the meninges are derived from mesenchymal cells. Thus, extradural meningiomas could arise in numerous unusual locations as a result of aberrant differentiation and/or misplacement of multipotent mesenchymal stem cells.[14]

CLINICAL PRESENTATION

Similar to many cranial and intracranial lesions, the clinical presentation and resulting differential diagnosis depend primarily on the location of the lesion. For example, calvarial intraosseous meningiomas most commonly present as slowly growing scalp masses, with possible relationship to a cranial suture.[15] These are typically firm and painless, with normal overlying skin, and may be detected incidentally.[16] Neurologic signs and symptoms are usually absent. In contrast, skull base intraosseous meningiomas may present with cranial nerve deficits, such as ophthalmoplegia or visual field problems, or signs and symptoms related to mass effect, such as proptosis. Symptoms, such as hearing loss, tinnitus, headache, and vague sensations in the head, are also reported.[4] One primary difference in clinical presentations between intradural and extradural intraosseous meningiomas is the potential for scalp involvement.

Extradural meningiomas, including intraosseous meningiomas, are reported to occur with the same frequency in each gender, unlike intradural meningiomas, which occur twice as frequently in women as in men.[16] Like intradural meningiomas, they predominantly occur later in life, but extradural meningiomas also have a second peak incidence during the second decade of life.[2] The tumors are nearly uniformly solitary, although 1 case report presented a patient with 2 separate lesions.

In this patient, an initial diagnosis of fibrous dysplasia was made after CT showed hyperostosis of the temporal and sphenoid bones. Two years later, a repeat CT scan showed the interval development of hyperostosis in the occipital bone and biopsy diagnosed intraosseous meningioma.[17]

RADIOGRAPHIC APPEARANCE

Like their dural based counterparts, intraosseous meningiomas may induce hyperostosis. In these cases, conventional radiographs demonstrate hyperdensity associated with the lesion, although superimposed bony structures may limit the usefulness of this radiographic modality. Skull radiographs can detect abnormalities in 30% to 60% of cases of intraosseous meningioma, including hyperostosis, thinning of bone, irregular foci of calcification, and atypical vascular markings.[6] Similarly, CT with bone windows shows a focally thickened, hyperdense, intradiploic lesion expanding the calvaria and destroying the cortical layers of the skull. The tumor is usually hyperdense on unenhanced CT, ranging from 65 to 85 Hounsfield units, and enhances densely after contrast administration similar to intradural meningiomas.[6] The expansion of bone and ground-glass appearance of this type of intraosseous meningioma may appear radiographically similar to fibrous dysplasia.[18] Differential diagnosis includes hyperostosis, Paget disease, fibrous sclerosis, sclerotic metastasis, and inflammatory lesions of bone.

Alternatively, primary intraosseous meningiomas may present as an osteolytic skull lesion.[11,16,19,20] It is thought that a majority of these meningiomas are osteoblastic (65%), with 35% osteolytic.[16] Similar expansion of the calvaria and cortical destruction is seen, although the intradiploic lesion is hypodense on plane films or CT. A report in 1995 reviewed the radiographic findings of the 34 published cases of intraosseous meningioma. Radiographic evidence of hyperostosis was noted in 20 (59%) cases, whereas 11 (35%) showed osteolytic changes in the surrounding bone. The remaining 2 cases (6%) revealed a mixed picture of both osteolysis and hyperostosis.[13] As of 2007, only 16 cases of the rare osteolytic subtype of intraosseous meningioma had been described in the literature, which represents less than 10% of reported cases overall.[11]

MRI findings are similar to those for intradural lesions and allow better delineation of tumors that have extracalvarial soft tissue extension. The tumors are typically hypointense on T1-weighted images and hyperintense on T2-weighted images. Prominent, homogeneous enhancement after gadolinium administration is typical. The tumors do not exhibit the dural tail often found with intradural meningiomas, but gadolinium enhancement of the underlying dura may be noted. This dural enhancement could be secondary to dural irritation or tumor invasion.[15]

A recent report evaluated angiographic findings of 10 patients with intraosseous meningioma. Consistent findings in a majority of patients included an enlarged, tortuous feeding artery, a dense tumor blush, and early venous drainage. Branches of the external carotid artery fed the tumor in most patients.[6]

Bone scintigraphy using technetium Tc 99m diphosphonate has been used to assess the response of an intraosseous meningioma to adjuvant therapy in a patient with an unresectable lesion.[4] Bone scintigraphy has also been used to demonstrate a tripling in size of an intraosseous meningioma over a 5-year period.[21]

DIFFERENTIAL DIAGNOSIS

Differential diagnosis is primarily based on radiographic appearance and clinical findings. Other lesions that can appear as a focal hyperdense skull lesion are eosinophilic granuloma, aneurysmal bone cyst, meningioma en plaque, osteoma, Paget disease, and fibrous dysplasia.[18,22] Fibrous dysplasia may be distinguished from intraosseous meningioma based on a patient's age. Fibrous dysplasia usually stops growing after puberty, whereas intraosseous meningiomas typically appear after puberty and continue to slowly grow. Also, fibrous dysplasia does not have a tumor blush on angiography that is typical of meningiomas.[6] Both fibrous dysplasia and intraosseous mengiomas expand bone and have a ground-glass appearance. Radiographically, however, the inner table of the skull looks smooth in fibrous dysplasia, whereas intraosseous meningiomas often demonstrate irregularity of the inner table, almost associated with a dural reaction.[18]

Meningioma en plaque may induce significant hyperostosis in the overlying bone, and tumor enhancement may be mistaken for dural reaction to an overlying intraosseous meningioma. Differential of these 2 entities may have intraoperative complications, because gross total removal of an intraosseous meningioma is critical for preventing long-term recurrence. On the other hand, hyperostotic bone induced by a meningioma may simply need to be removed for decompression, but gross total removal not necessary.

Clinically, slow-growing skull lesions with normal overlying skin may include intraosseous hemangioma, giant cell tumor, aneurysmal bone cyst, fibrous dysplasia, and eosinophilic granuloma.[23] Lesions, however, such as aneurysmal bone cyst and dermoid, can typically be distinguished on imaging.

Osteolytic intraosseous meningiomas may appear similar to other lesions, such as hemangioma, hemangiopericytoma, epidermoid tumor, dermoid, brown tumor, multiple myeloma, plasmacytoma, giant cell tumor, osteogenic sarcoma, eosinophilic granuloma, and metastatic cancer.[11,16,20]

HISTOPATHOLOGY

Intraoperative pathologic examination may be limited, especially in cases of hyperostosis present, due to the presence of bone throughout the specimen. In these cases, decalcification of the specimen is required prior to histopathologic assessment. Microscopic pathology often reveals findings pathognomonic for intradural meningiomas, including psammoma bodies and eosinophilic tumor cells with indistinct borders and nuclear pseudoinclusions grouped in a whorl pattern.[4,5,18] The bone may appear normal, with replacement of the marrow by fat, fibrosis, and tumor cells. The cells are usually meningothelial in origin. Histopathologic examination of intraosseous meningiomas may reveal an unusual subtype. For example, a chordoid type intraosseous meningioma was described that demonstrated regions of eosinophilic cells contained in a mucous-rich matrix. This histopathologic pattern was similar to, and could, therefore, be confused with, chordoma.[10] Consistent with their intradural counterparts, immunostaining of tumor cells of intraosseous meningiomas is usually positive for vimentin.[5]

Although intraosseous meningiomas are largely described as slow-growing, benign lesion, recent literature indicates that calvarial meningiomas have higher incidence of malignant features than intradural meningiomas (11% vs 2%).[24–26] This may be reflected by microscopic tumor invasion of underlying dura or overlying soft tissue structures. One lesion, described histologically as atypical, was found to secrete carcinoembryonic antigen.[25]

NOMENCLATURE AND CLASSIFICATION

Until recently, a unifying classification scheme for meningiomas that arise in locations other than the dura has been lacking. In the literature, meningiomas that arise in locations other than the subdural compartment are given a variety of names. These include ectopic, secondary, extracalvarial, cutaneous, extracranial, primary extraneuraxial, and extradural.[16,18] Extradural meningiomas that arise in the skull have been referred to as calvarial, intradiploic, and intraosseous.[5] Another difficulty with nomenclature in the literature is that PIMs that grow through the bone or metastasize have occasionally been misnamed for their secondary location.

A recent case series offered a unifying nomenclature to reduce confusion caused by the variety of terms in the literature.[2] The term, *primary extradural meningioma (PEM)*, differentiates tumors that arise separate from dura from those that originate in the dura but have extracranial extension. This name also differentiates these tumors from extracranial meningiomas that represent distant metastases from PIMs. Another issue arises when cells from a presumed extradural meningioma invade the dura mater.[15,16] Depending on the radiographic appearance and surgical findings, these tumors may be difficult to definitively classify.[11] Other investigators maintain that dural invasion precludes a diagnosis of intraosseous meningioma.[6]

The following illustrates the classification scheme for PEMs developed by Lang and colleagues.[2] Tumors that are purely extracalvarial are type I, purely calvarial tumors are type II, and calvarial tumors with extracalvarial extension are type III. Each category is further divided into convexity (C) or skull base (B) subtypes based on anatomic location. Thus, intraosseous meningiomas could be considered type II or type III PEMs based on whether extracalvarial extension is observed.

Difficulties with nomenclature discrepancies in the literature were addressed in a report by Lang and colleagues.[2] Additional consideration could be given for further distinguishing intraosseous meningiomas based on the radiographic changes observed in the bone involved with the tumor. Previous reports suggested that intraosseous meningiomas that presented with the clinical and radiographic picture of scalp swelling, osteolytic skull lesion, and extracranial soft tissue mass were more suspicious for malignant meningiomas. For example, a case series reported 3 patients who presented with this clinical triad, all of whom were ultimately diagnosed with malignant meningiomas.[26] Other case reports also described histologically malignant or atypical intraosseous meningiomas in patients who presented with an osteolytic lesion and soft tissue mass.[24,25]

TREATMENT

Surgical treatment with wide excision of the lesion, if possible, is potentially curative.[4] Ideally, cranial reconstruction occurs as part of the same

procedure.[16] Lesions of the skull base may not be completely resected, in which case decompression of vital neural structures is performed. The use of neuronavigation for preoperative planning and intraoperative surgical navigation may facilitate maximal resection of the tumor. Additionally, preoperative assessment of potential defect geometry, for example, with 3-D CT, may allow implantation of a custom-made cranioplasty implant at the time of resection.[27] Angiography to rule out vascular involvement has been reported, although embolization was not performed.[18]

Postoperative imaging is important for evaluating the extent of resection and monitoring for tumor recurrence or progress. The term, *intraosseous meningiomas*, denotes tumors that originate in the bones of the calvarium or skull base. Although histologically benign, these tumors may encroach on or involve certain parts of the skull that render the lesion not completely resectable. Tumors that cannot be completely resected that are histologically benign and neurologically asymptomatic may be followed with serial imaging. Also, as discussed previously, 11% of tumors may have evidence of malignant changes. Patients with such lesions may be considered for adjuvant therapy, depending on clinical circumstances. Adjuvant therapy may be considered in cases of patients with unresectable tumors causing neurologic deficit or that demonstrate malignant or atypical features histologically. This may include radiation therapy, such as external beam or Gamma Knife treatment; chemotherapy with cytotoxic agents, such as BCNU; and hormonal therapy.

Previous publications recommended adjuvant radiation therapy for patients with lesions that are not completely resectable in whom the residual lesion is symptomatic or shows radiographic evidence of progression.[13] Other case reports describe postoperative radiotherapy without indicating the extent of tumor resection.[17]

A recent report described the use of etidronate disodium to treat an inoperable, biopsy-proved intraosseous meningioma. The tumor involved the sagittal sinus and was associated with significant hyperostosis. The patient received etidronate, 200 mg/d, for 6 months. This resulted in amelioration of the patient's presenting symptom (tinnitus) and reduction in tracer accumulation on serial bone scintigraphy studies.[4]

SUMMARY

Intraosseous meningiomas are rare lesions that originate in the skull and represent the most common type of extradural meningioma. The lesions are often asymptomatic but can cause proptosis and neurologic symptoms depending on their size and location. Radiographic and clinical presentations generate diagnostic suspicion that may assist with preoperative planning. A majority of these tumors cause hyperostosis that may mimic fibrous dysplasia. Although most are benign, osteolytic lesions are more likely malignant.

Intraosseous meningiomas likely originate from entrapment of arachnoid cells within the bone. Multiple theories exist on how the cells become located in the skull, although none is universally accepted and separate etiologies are possible. The treatment of choice is surgical resection, which is potentially curative. Using 3-D neuronavigation and operative planning, tumor resection and cranioplasty may be performed simultaneously. Tumors that cannot be completely resected may require consideration for adjuvant therapy. This may include radiation therapy, chemotherapy, and/or etidronate. Further work is required, however, to elucidate any optimal adjuvant therapy regimens.

REFERENCES

1. Hoye SJ, Hoar CS Jr, Murray JE. Extracranial meningioma presenting as a tumor of the neck. Am J Surg 1960;100:486–9.

2. Lang FF, Macdonald OK, Fuller GN, et al. Primary extradural meningiomas: a report on nine cases and review of the literature from the era of computerized tomography scanning. J Neurosurg 2000;93: 940–50.

3. Muzumdar DP, Vengsarkar US, Bhatjiwale MG, et al. Diffuse calvarial meningioma: a case report. J Postgrad Med 2001;47:116–8.

4. Inagaki K, Otsuka F, Matsui T, et al. Effect of etidronate on intraosseous meningioma. Endocr J 2004; 51:389–90.

5. Cirak B, Guven MB, Ugras S, et al. Fronto-orbito-nasal intradiploic meningioma in a child. Pediatr Neurosurg 2000;32:48–51.

6. Changhong L, Naiyin C, Yuehuan G, et al. Primary intraosseous meningiomas of the skull. Clin Radiol 1997;52:546–9.

7. Pompili A, Caroli F, Cattani F, et al. Intradiploic meningioma of the orbital roof. Neurosurgery 1983;12: 565–8.

8. Azar-Kia B, Sarwar M, Marc JA, et al. Intraosseous meningioma. Neuroradiology 1974;6:246–53.

9. Devi B, Bhat D, Madhusudhan H, et al. Primary intraosseous meningioma of orbit and anterior cranial fossa: a case report and literature review. Australas Radiol 2001;45:211–4.

10. Van Tassel P, Lee YY, Ayala A, et al. Case report 680. Intraosseous meningioma of the sphenoid bone. Skeletal Radiol 1991;20:383–6.

11. Agrawal V, Ludwig N, Agrawal A, et al. Intraosseous intracranial meningioma. AJNR Am J Neuroradiol 2007;28:314–5.

12. Turner OA, Laird AT. Meningioma with traumatic etiology. Report of a case. J Neurosurg 1966;24:96–8.

13. Crawford TS, Kleinschmidt-DeMasters BK, Lillehei KO. Primary intraosseous meningioma. Case report. J Neurosurg 1995;83:912–5.

14. Lopez DA, Silvers DN, Helwig EB. Cutaneous meningiomas–a clinicopathologic study. Cancer 1974; 34:728–44.

15. Arana E, Diaz C, Latorre FF, et al. Primary intraosseous meningiomas. Acta Radiol 1996;37:937–42.

16. Tokgoz N, Oner YA, Kaymaz M, et al. Primary intraosseous meningioma: CT and MRI appearance. AJNR Am J Neuroradiol 2005;26(8):2053–6.

17. El Mahou S, Popa L, Constantin A, et al. Laroche M. multiple intraosseous meningiomas. Clin Rheumatol 2006;25:553–4.

18. Daffner RH, Yakulis R, Maroon JC. Intraosseous meningioma. Skeletal Radiol 1998;27:108–11.

19. Levin M, Wertheim SE, Klein E, et al. Unusual lytic intraosseous meningioma. J Neuroimaging 1995;5: 247–8.

20. Rosahl SK, Mirzayan MJ, Samii M. Osteolytic intraosseous meningiomas: illustrated review. Acta Neurochir (Wien) 2004;146:1245–9.

21. Kanmaz B, Weissman DE, Akansel G, et al. Intraosseous meningioma: appearance on bone scintigraphy over five years. J Nucl Med 1993;34:961–2.

22. Jayaraj K, Martinez S, Freeman A, et al. Intraosseous meningioma–a mimicry of Paget's disease? J Bone Miner Res 2001;16:1154–6.

23. Politi M, Romeike BF, Papanagiotou P, et al. Intraosseous hemangioma of the skull with dural tail sign: radiologic features with pathologic correlation. AJNR Am J Neuroradiol 2005;26:2049–52.

24. Husaini TA. An unusual osteolytic meningioma. J Pathol 1970;101:57–8.

25. Partington MD, Scheithauer BW, Piepgras DG. Carcinoembryonic antigen production associated with an osteolytic meningioma. Case report. J Neurosurg 1995;82:489–92.

26. Younis G, Sawaya R. Intracranial osteolytic malignant meningiomas appearing as extracranial soft-tissue masses. Neurosurgery 1992;30:932–5.

27. Westendorff C, Kaminsky J, Ernemann U, et al. Image-guided sphenoid wing meningioma resection and simultaneous computer-assisted Cranio-Orbital reconstruction: technical case report. Neurosurgery 2007;60:E173–4.

Management of Spinal Meningiomas

Vijay M. Ravindra, MD, MSPH, Meic H. Schmidt, MD, MBA*

KEYWORDS

- Spinal meningioma • Atypical • Myelopathy • Intraoperative monitoring

KEY POINTS

- Spinal meningiomas are benign tumors that account for approximately 1.2% to 12.7% of all meningiomas and 25% of all spinal cord tumors.
- The treatment Is surgical, with the primary goal to achieve complete tumor removal while minimizing neurologic dysfunction.
- Radiotherapy can be considered for recurrent for challenging surgical cases and for patients with higher-grade histopathology (World Health Organization grade II or III), but it remains an adjuvant therapy for spinal cord meningiomas.
- Emerging molecular and genetic targets may represent adjuvant treatment options for both surgical and nonsurgical treatment.

 Video content accompanies this article at http://www.neurosurgery.theclinics.com

INTRODUCTION

Spinal meningiomas are the most common spinal tumors in adult patients, and they are typically managed with surgery to achieve a gross total resection when possible while minimizing neurologic dysfunction. The first case of successful surgical resection of a spinal meningioma was performed by Victor Horsley more than a century ago.[1] Advances in surgical techniques and adjuvant treatment modalities have further improved the opportunities to achieve a cure.

Epidemiology

Intradural spinal tumors have an incidence of 64 per 100,000 person-years and account for 3% of primary central nervous system (CNS) tumors.[2] Spinal meningiomas are intradural, extramedullary lesions (**Fig. 1**) that arise from meningothelial arachnoid gap cells within the spinal dura mater.

Spinal intradural-extramedullary tumors account for two-thirds of all intraspinal neoplasms,[3] and spinal meningiomas are the second most common intradural spine tumor after neuromas.[4] As the most common spinal tumor in adults, they account for up to 45% of intradural spinal tumors but only 6.5% of overall craniospinal tumors In adults.[2,4] Intracranial meningiomas are much more prevalent than spinal meningiomas, which account for only 1.2% to 12.7% of all meningiomas[5] and 25% of all spinal tumors.[5–7]

The peak age of occurrence for spinal meningiomas is 40 to 70 years.[5] Spinal meningiomas most commonly affect middle-aged women, with a greater disparity of women to men than is seen with intracranial meningiomas. In one series, the female:male ratio was as high as 4:1.[8] This preponderance in women is thought to arise from tissue response to sex hormones and subsequent growth.[5,9] Although the effect of sex hormones

Disclosures: None.
Department of Neurosurgery, Clinical Neurosciences Center, University of Utah, 175 N. Medical Drive East, Salt Lake City, UT 84132, USA
* Corresponding author. Department of Neurosurgery, Clinical Neurosciences Center, University of Utah, 175 North Medical Drive East, Salt Lake City, UT 84132.
E-mail address: neuropub@hsc.utah.edu

Neurosurg Clin N Am 27 (2016) 195–205
http://dx.doi.org/10.1016/j.nec.2015.11.010
1042-3680/16/$ – see front matter © 2016 Elsevier Inc. All rights reserved.

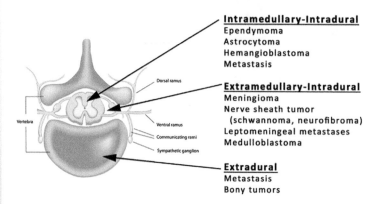

Intramedullary-Intradural
Ependymoma
Astrocytoma
Hemangioblastoma
Metastasis

Extramedullary-Intradural
Meningioma
Nerve sheath tumor
(schwannoma, neurofibroma)
Leptomeningeal metastases
Medulloblastoma

Extradural
Metastasis
Bony tumors

Dorsal ramus

Vertebra

Ventral ramus

Communicating rami

Sympathetic ganglion

Fig. 1. Illustration showing the intradural, extramedullary location of spinal meningiomas as well as other spinal cord tumors. (*Courtesy of* Fotosearch, with permission. © Fotosearch.com.)

on meningiomas is suspected, several other receptor types may play a role in pathogenesis, including[9] the following:

- Steroid receptors
- Peptidergic receptors
- Growth factor receptors
- Aminergic receptors

Most spinal meningiomas are histologically benign or World Health Organization (WHO) grade I; however, a small percentage are atypical (WHO grade II) or anaplastic (WHO grade III).[7,10,11] The histologic subtypes are similar to those seen in cranial meningiomas, including the following:

- Meningothelial (WHO grade I)
- Metaplastic (WHO grade I)
- Psammomatous (WHO grade I)
- Transitional (mixed) (WHO grade I)
- Atypical (WHO grade II)
- Clear cell (WHO grade II)
- Anaplastic (WHO grade III).

The psammomatous (WHO grade I), meningothelial (WHO grade I), and transitional (WHO grade I) subtypes are the most common histologic subtypes seen in spinal meningiomas. Overall, spinal meningiomas show a lower recurrence rate than intracranial meningiomas.[7,10,12] This is most likely a reflection of their less aggressive histopathology. When comparing the outcomes of surgical resection among the subtypes, patients with psammomatous pathology have been shown to have worse neurologic outcomes.[12] Malignant transformation of spinal meningiomas, although rare, occurs in approximately 3% of cases.[10]

Spinal meningiomas may present with or lead to acute or chronic spinal cord compression, neurologic dysfunction, and progressive myelopathy, depending on location. Because spinal meningiomas grow slowly, neurologic deficits are the result of significant spinal cord compression. Patients most commonly present with the following:

- Pain
- Sensory loss
- Weakness
- Sphincter disturbances

Although serious neurologic deficits may be a result of these tumors, surgical treatment is often curative, with few complications and rapid functional recovery.[5,8,13–15] Advances in radiological and surgical technique (eg, MRI, neuromonitoring, intraoperative ultrasonography, microsurgery, and ultrasonic surgical aspirator) have resulted in earlier diagnosis and the ability to achieve gross total resection.[8]

Patients with spinal meningioma can be assessed and graded on neurologic dysfunction using the McCormick scale (**Table 1**).[16]

Although the diagnosis of spinal meningioma may be highly suspected based on imaging characteristics or previous clinical information (eg, recurrence, history of neurofibromatosis), tissue diagnosis and confirmation is needed in many cases.

Surgical Management

Surgery is the definitive treatment for symptomatic spinal meningiomas and provides the possibility for total resection and cure.[17] The outcomes of surgical treatment for spinal meningiomas are mostly favorable[5,6,8,13–15,18–20]; however, individual outcome is dependent on the size and location of the tumor and the preoperative neurologic state of the patient. Although originally applied to intracranial meningiomas, the Simpson grading classification[21] is commonly used to define and describe the extent of resection for spinal meningiomas (see Surgical approach section).

Table 1
McCormick scale for neurologic dysfunction in patients with spinal meningioma

Grade	Definition
0	No symptoms or neurologic deficits
1	Neurologically normal, mild focal deficit not significantly affecting function of involved limbs; mild spasticity or reflex abnormality; normal gait
2	Presence of sensorimotor deficit affecting function of involved limb; mild to moderate gait difficulty; severe pain or dysesthetic syndrome impairing patient's quality of life; patient still functions and ambulates independently
3	More severe neurologic deficit; requires cane/brace for ambulation of significant bilateral upper extremity impairment; may or may not function independently
4	Severe deficit; requires wheelchair or cane/brace with bilateral upper extremity impairment; usually not independent

Adapted from McCormick PC, Torres R, Post KD, et al. Intramedullary ependymoma of the spinal cord. J Neurosurg 1990;72(4):524.

Genetic and Molecular Markers

Genetic and molecular targets for meningioma therapy are becoming more commonplace. Historically, spinal meningiomas and intracranial meningiomas have been treated similarly, but recent genetic information may change this paradigm.

Multiple genes have been implicated with spinal meningiomas. Several studies have reported a deletion of chromosome 22q and the associated gene NF2 in cases of spinal meningioma.[21,22] One study using data from DNA microarray found that, in addition to a greater association with psammomatous and transitional subtypes, spinal meningiomas had greater likelihood than intracranial meningiomas of chromosome 22 deletion.[22] In fact, complete or partial loss of chromosome 22 has been demonstrated in more than 50% of patients with spinal meningiomas.[21,23] For instance, Ketter and colleagues[23] demonstrated that each of 23 patients with spinal meningiomas had a normal chromosomal set or a monosomy of chromosome 22. Interestingly, this genotype was not associated with disease recurrence, whereas, in contrast, intracranial meningiomas have a direct correlation between multiple chromosomal aberrations and higher rates of recurrence.

Spinal meningiomas can have complete or partial loss of chromosome 22, along with loss of 1p, 9p, and 10q with the gain of 5p and 17q when compared with the chromosome complement in the patient's own lymphocytes.[21] These changes are most commonly seen in atypical and anaplastic subtypes. Additionally, spinal meningiomas likely originate from a single cell clone versus a collection of cells; 35 of 1555 genes were more highly expressed in spinal meningiomas than in intracranial tumors,[22] including those involved in the following:

- Transcription: *Hox* genes, *NR4* family of genes, *KLF4, FOSL2,* and *TCF 8*
- Intracellular signaling: *RGS16, DUSP5, DUSP1, SOCS3,* and *CMKOR*
- Extracellular signaling: *L6, TGFB1I4, CYR61,* and *CDH2*

Other genes that have been implicated in spinal meningioma development include the following:

- Matrix metalloproteinase-9 (MMP-9)[24], which functions in protein upregulation involved in cell growth and invasion
- *SMARCE1*[25], which is involved in regulation of secondary DNA structure within chromosomes and is associated with multiple spinal meningioma formation.

The gene mutations found in intracranial meningiomas (*DAL1, TIMP, p16, p15, p14ARF, NDRG2, ADTB1, DLC1, c-myc, bcl-2,* and *STAT3*) have not been fully evaluated in spinal meningioma.[26] Although there is limited information, further study of these and other genes may provide further insight into molecular and genetic targets for therapy.[27]

Tumor Locations

Spinal meningiomas can occur anywhere along the spinal cord. The most commonly reported location is the thoracic spine (67%–84%), followed by the cervical spine (14%–27%), and the lumbar spine (2%–14%).[5,6,8,13–15,18]

Previous studies have shown that patients 50 years or younger have a higher frequency of spinal meningiomas in the cervical spine (39%), with most occurring in the upper cervical spine.[28] Levy and colleagues[6] reported that tumor location varied by sex, with a preponderance of thoracic spine meningiomas appearing in female patients. In addition to location in the spine, the location in relation to the spinal cord (lateral [68%], posterior [18%], or anterior [15%]) is also commonly used to describe spinal meningiomas.[6] There are no other specific patterns recognized to be associated with location, thus thorough imaging workup and evaluation are needed to fully ascertain the origin and location of these lesions. As described previously (see **Fig. 1**), spinal meningiomas are traditionally described as intradural, extramedullary lesions, although 5% to 14% of spinal meningiomas may have an extradural component[5,6,13–15,18]; additionally, there are case reports of entirely extradural meningiomas.[5,14,15] The presence of multiple spinal cord meningiomas has been reported as well, but this is a rare occurrence.

PATIENT EVALUATION OVERVIEW

When evaluating patients with suspected spinal cord lesions, it is important to obtain a full history and physical and a detailed neurologic examination. Patients will most commonly present with delayed onset of neurologic symptoms. Multiple previous studies have indicated that patients report symptom duration lasting an average of 1 to 2 years before initial presentation.[6,14,15,18] This, however, can be contrasted to patients who may have long-standing pain (>2 years), radiculopathy, or weakness secondary to the lesion. Typically, back or radicular pain precedes weakness and sensory disturbances, with sphincter dysfunction usually as a late finding.[8]

Advancements in imaging techniques and resolution have improved the diagnostics in evaluating suspected spinal cord lesions. Previously, the differential diagnosis for suspected spinal cord lesion included the following[6,13]:

- Multiple sclerosis
- Syringomyelia
- Pernicious anemia
- Herniated nucleus pulposus.

MRI is currently the best imaging modality for diagnosing spinal cord lesions because it offers markedly increased sensitivity and specificity, especially for spinal cord meningiomas. Before the widespread use of MRI, computed tomography myelography was used for diagnosing spinal cord meningiomas. The use of MRI for diagnosis has led to improved detection an average of 6 months earlier,[18] which in turn has led to improved neurologic function at the time of diagnosis. On MRI, spinal meningiomas are isointense to the normal spinal cord on T1-weighted and T2-weighted images; they also characteristically display intense, homogeneous contrast enhancement after intravenous administration of gadolinium.[13] **Fig. 2** represents an algorithm that can be used when evaluating patients with suspected spinal cord meningiomas. The differential diagnosis, which can be narrowed to tumors based on MRI findings, but still may require surgical biopsy for definitive diagnosis, includes the following:

- Metastatic lesion
- Dropped metastatic lesion from intracranial disease
- Primary CNS tumor (glioma, astrocytoma)
- Schwannoma
- Neurofibroma

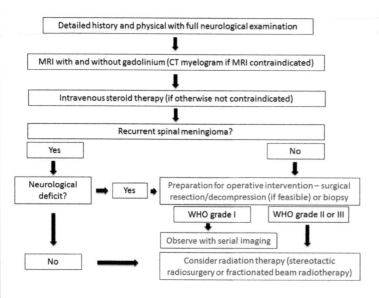

Fig. 2. Algorithm for evaluating patients with suspected spinal cord meningioma.

- Lipoma
- Malignant peripheral nerve sheath tumor

SURGICAL APPROACH

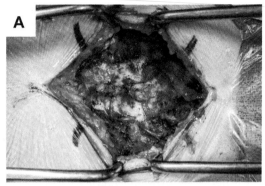

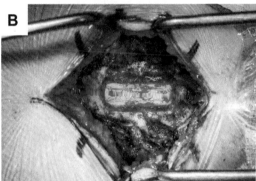

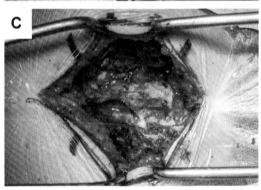

The treatment for spinal meningiomas includes surgical excision to confirm histologic diagnosis and decompression of the neural elements. Although minimally invasive resection of intradural-extramedullary spinal tumors has been described,[29] the most commonly reported surgical procedure is a single-level posterior laminectomy for access to the thecal sac and spinal cord for tumor resection; however, laminoplasty or multilevel laminectomy with or without spinal fusion are additional surgical options (**Fig. 3**). To minimize the extent of bony opening, particularly in the thoracic spine, fluoroscopy can be used to identify a radiopaque marker placed preoperatively to aid with intraoperative localization.[30] In cases in which there is ventral extension or origin of the spinal meningioma, removal of the articular process laterally may be necessary to provide a corridor to the ventral spinal cord.

For meningiomas located in the ventral or ventrolateral cervical spinal cord, an anterior cervical approach with corpectomy followed by grafting and fusion may provide an adequate corridor for tumor resection; however, primary dural repair may be difficult in this scenario, making cerebrospinal fluid (CSF) diversion necessary. For lesions located in the lateral or anterior corridor located between T3 and L2, a lateral extracavitary approach can be used to allow for circumferential neural decompression with direct visualization and extrapleural/extravisceral dissection.[31] This approach may require posterior stabilization in the setting of extensive pedicle removal and disruption of the ipsilateral facet joint.

Costotransversectomy also can be used to provide surgical access to ventral and ventrolateral pathology via a posterior approach.[32] Partial laminectomy and facetectomy is performed, but fusion may not be necessary unless there is violation of the anterior column structures. In addition to the complication profile for any spinal tumor, injury to the great vessels and to the radicular arteries leading to spinal cord infarct can also result from the use of this approach.[32]

The use of spinal fusion in the setting of spinal meningioma surgery depends on the dimensions of the lesion, location along the spinal axis, position in the spinal cord, and the presence of extradural or spinal extension.[33] Predictors of spinal instability after spinal tumor resection include multilevel laminectomy, disruption of the facet joints, and corpectomy.[34–36] Meningiomas at the

Fig. 3. (A) Intraoperative photograph demonstrating the bony exposure needed to perform a single or multilevel laminectomy for resection. (B) Photograph showing laminectomy and exposure of the dural surface. (C) Intraoperative photograph demonstrating 2-level laminoplasty after spinal meningioma resection.

occipitocervical junction and cervicothoracic and thoracolumbar regions are at higher risk for instability with treatment because of the transitional change in the axis of motion and mobility occurring at these locations[36–38]; thus, short-segment stabilization may be required. Misra and Morgan[33] previously suggested a classification scheme of bony removal for spinal meningiomas and the relationship between the approach and need for stabilization. Decisions to perform spinal fusion, however, should be made on a case-by-case basis considering the exposure necessary for tumor resection, bony removal, and potential ligamentous disruption in relation to mobility, biomechanics, and patient comfort.

Despite advances in surgical technique and neurologic monitoring, surgical resection of spinal cord tumors still poses a significant challenge to neurosurgeons.[39] The most significant risk is postoperative neurologic worsening, including, but not limited to, motor weakness, sensory loss, and autonomic dysfunction. Although steps are taken to mitigate neurologic damage, some risk remains. Use of the operating microscope to perform resection has become the standard of care. The use of stereotactic navigation for spinal cord tumors has not become as commonplace as it has for intracranial lesions; however, intraoperative ultrasonography can be a useful adjunct in the identification and localization of meningiomas by providing information about size, shape, and degree of displacement of the spinal cord.[40]

The goal of surgery is to minimize displacement and manipulation of the spinal cord by using an adequately wide exposure to make the tumor and its associated dural attachment accessible.[8] This can be accomplished through separation of the dentate ligament(s). After the arachnoid plane is developed to access the tumor, resection of the tumor is undertaken (Video 1).

Spinal meningiomas are firm, encapsulated lesions with an identifiable dural attachment (**Fig. 4**). Most commonly they grossly appear purple or yellow in appearance; however, this may vary based on histologic subtype. The tumor is internally debulked using bipolar electrocautery, gentle suction, ultrasonic surgical aspirator, microscissors, or the laser.[8] As the tumor becomes free from the spinal cord, it is rolled away from the spinal cord toward its dural attachment. This can be difficult in cases of spinal meningiomas with significant ventral extension or a ventral attachment. Once the dural attachment is identified and transected, the attempt is made to eliminate dura with remaining tumor.

Although the Simpson classification[41] was originally applied to intracranial meningiomas, it has been used to describe and define the extent of resection for spinal meningiomas as well (**Table 2**).

In most published series, the dural attachment of spinal meningiomas is cauterized rather than resected because of the variable location of the dural attachment and the difficulty of repairing a dural defect in the anterior and lateral corridor. An additional technique involves separation of the dura into its inner and outer leaflets to allow resection of the tumor from the inner leaflet and closure of the outer leaflet primarily. It has recently been

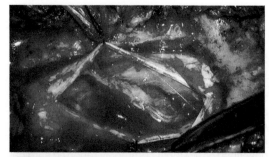
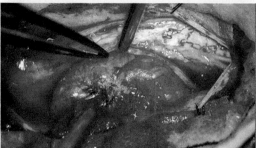
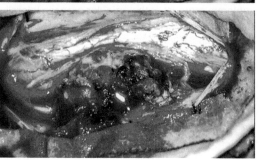

Fig. 4. Intraoperative photographs after dural opening identifying the spinal meningioma, which grossly appears purple in appearance with evidence of a firm capsule and definitive plane between the dura and tumor.

Table 2
Simpson classification of resection for spinal meningiomas

Grade	Definition
1	Macroscopically complete removal of tumor with excision of its dural attachment
2	Macroscopically complete removal of tumor with coagulation of its dural attachment
3	Macroscopically complete removal of tumor, without resection or coagulation of its dural attachment
4	Partial removal, leaving tumor in situ

Adapted from Simpson D. The recurrence of intracranial meningiomas after surgical treatment. J Neurol Neurosurg Psychiatry 1957;20(1):24–5.

shown that Simpson grade I–III resection is associated with symptom resolution and low recurrence rates for atypical meningiomas.[17] After tumor resection is completed, the durotomy is primarily closed, when possible, using a running 4-0 Nurolon suture (**Fig. 5**).

With a wide variability in location, surgical resectability is not a generalized concept. Spinal meningiomas that are anterior, en plaque, recurrent tumors with scarring, and meningiomas with calcification are considered barriers to total resection.[5,6,14,15,18] Tumors with these characteristics require careful surgical planning that may require CSF diversion, adjuvant therapy, and close imaging surveillance.

Neuromonitoring

Neuromonitoring is used to reduce and minimize the likelihood of postoperative neurologic deficits during surgery for spinal cord meningiomas. Neuromonitoring can provide information regarding the following[14]:

- Extent of tissue manipulation and resection
- Preservation of function

The 2 most commonly used techniques are transcranial motor evoked potential (Tc-MEP) and somatosensory evoked potentials (SSEP) monitoring.

Tc-MEPs, which have been used for intraoperative monitoring for more than 20 years, are the most commonly used because of their widespread availability and the approval of the techniques by the US Food and Drug Administration.[42,43] Tc-MEP involves applying a train of high-voltage stimuli to electrodes on the surface of the head to activate motor pathways and produce either a

motor contraction (muscle MEP) or a nerve action potential (D-wave) that can be recorded.[44] This information can be used intraoperatively to ascertain the condition of the motor tracts being manipulated during tumor surgery.[44] This mode of monitoring is most useful for tumors located in a location that is[14]

- Anterior
- Anterolateral
- Compressing the corticospinal tract

SSEP was the first modality used for monitoring the function of the spinal cord during surgical manipulation.[45] SSEP involves stimulation of peripheral nerves in the upper and lower extremities. In the upper extremity, the impulses are conducted from the peripheral nerve to the spinal cord and brachial plexus, where the Erb point potential is generated, which synapses in the dorsal column nuclei, giving the N13 potential. The fibers then pass via the medial lemniscus to reach the thalamus, where the N20 potential is generated. After arriving at the primary sensory cortex, the N20 and P22 potentials are generated.[44] In the lower extremity, the SSEP travels past the popliteal fossa, generating a popliteal potential, before reaching the lumbosacral plexus.[44] As the impulses enter the cauda equina, N21, a lumbar potential, is generated.[44] SSEP monitoring is most useful for tumors located in a location that is[14]

- Posterior
- Posterolateral
- Compressing the dorsal column pathways

Additional modalities commonly used in spinal surgery include spontaneous and stimulated electromyography, direct spinal cord stimulation, and reflex monitoring.[44] Choice of monitoring technique, findings, and effects of anesthesia should be considered by the surgeon.

SURGICAL COMPLICATIONS

Most perioperative morbidity is related to the extent of manipulation of the surrounding spinal cord structures. Each patient's preoperative functional status is highly correlated to his or her postoperative functional status. Overall, the mortality rate from surgical intervention of spinal meningiomas is low, ranging from 0% to 3%. In all reported cases of death, the cause is unrelated to the spinal meningioma. There is a risk of CSF leak, ranging from 0% to 4%,[8] which may necessitate CSF diversion or prolonged bed rest depending on the location of the meningioma and

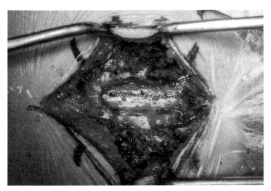

Fig. 5. Intraoperative photograph demonstrating primary dural closure following spinal meningioma resection with a running 4-0 Nurolon suture. Closure should be performed in a watertight fashion to prevent CSF leak.

dural opening. Potential postoperative complications include the following:

- Pulmonary embolism
- Hematoma (either subdural or epidural)
- Pneumonia: hospital or community acquired
- Myocardial infarction
- Deep venous thrombosis

FUNCTIONAL AND NEUROLOGIC OUTCOME

The functional and neurologic outcomes for spinal meningiomas are quite good. Emphasis must be placed on careful documentation and monitoring of the preoperative and postoperative neurologic examinations. The Frankel Scale may be used to provide common language[46] for grading functional disturbance of daily life activities and gait disturbances (**Table 3**).

In a series of 130 patients, Sandalcioglu and colleagues[7] reported an improved or unchanged neurologic function in 126 patients (96%), with worsening in 4 patients (3%). Similar findings have been demonstrated previously, with functional improvement occurring in up to 95% of cases, with neurologic deterioration in fewer than 10%.[5,6,13–15,18] In fact, patients with severe neurologic deficits preoperatively may exhibit full recovery after surgical resection followed by intensive rehabilitation.[6,18] Transient worsening in neurologic functioning of typically no more than 6 months has been demonstrated in some cases and is thought to be secondary to surgical manipulation and vasogenic edema[5,15,18]; however, this finding has not been reported since the widespread utilization of the intraoperative microscope began. Sandalcioglu and colleagues[7] found

several risk factors that led to neurologic deterioration, including the following:

- Patients between the ages of 76 and 80 years
- Complete calcification of the tumor (based on intraoperative inspection)

Interestingly, they found no association between the location of the dural attachment, tumor extension, or resection grade and postoperative neurologic deterioration.[7]

SPINAL MENINGIOMA RECURRENCE

The recurrence of spinal meningiomas is quite low, reported from 1.3% to 6.4%.[5,6,13–15] In general, spinal meningiomas are more benign than intracranial meningiomas. This is attributable to the more indolent nature of spinal meningiomas and is most likely due to the lack of genetic abnormalities that are often found in recurrent intracranial meningiomas.[23] In addition, the slow growth rate and propensity for spinal meningiomas to present in patients later in life also contributes to the lower recurrence rate.[8]

Although the overall recurrence rate is quite low for spinal cord meningiomas, the following subset of patients tend to have recurrence[18]:

- Patients with en plaque or infiltrative meningiomas
- Patients with partially resected lesions

In contrast to intracranial meningiomas, spinal meningiomas do not have a correlation between recurrence and excision of the dural attachment.[5,13,14,18] In their large series, Cohen-Gadol and colleagues[28] found that recurrence rates were higher in patients younger than 50 years because of a higher frequency of cervical spine meningiomas, extradural tumor extension, and en plaque growth, all of which are barriers to complete resection and implicate a more difficult initial operation.

PHARMACOLOGIC TREATMENT OPTIONS

There are previous reports of the use of hydroxyurea, interferon-alpha 2B, and octreotide to treat refractory, high-grade intracranial meningiomas. In addition, for intracranial meningiomas, current and future targets include cytotoxic agents, hormonal agents, immunomodulators, growth factor specific targets, and others.[47] Although there is a paucity of similar information on spinal meningiomas, there is hope that elucidation of molecular biomarkers and genetics may target specific therapy in the future. Given the propensity for these patients to present with pain or neurologic

Table 3 Frankel scale	
Frankel Grade	**Definition**
A.	No motor or sensory function below the level of injury
B.	Some preserved sensory function
C.	Some preserved motor function, unable to walk
D.	Preserved useful motor function, able to walk
E.	Normal motor and sensory function

Adapted from Frankel HL, Hancock DO, Hyslop G, et al. The value of postural reduction in the initial management of closed injuries of the spine with paraplegia and tetraplegia. I. Paraplegia 1969;7(3):182.

dysfunction, however, surgical decompression with a goal of gross total resection continues to be the standard treatment.

ADJUVANT RADIOTHERAPY AND RADIOSURGERY

The treatment for spinal cord meningiomas is primarily surgical, although radiotherapy may be used as an adjunct for subtotal resection or recurrence. The role for radiotherapy after subtotal resection is not fully understood, given that spinal meningiomas have been shown to have an indolent course.[13,15] Radiotherapy has been suggested to be useful after subtotal excision in cases of recurrent spinal meningiomas or as an alternative primary treatment when operative intervention carries an elevated risk because of tumor location or patient comorbidities.[6,13,15] Radiotherapy may be reserved for patients with grade III spinal meningiomas or grade II spinal meningiomas after recurrence or subtotal resection.[48,49] Recently, Sun and colleagues[17] demonstrated that patients with WHO grade II histology may not require adjuvant radiotherapy after surgery and, more importantly, that gross total resection without adjuvant radiotherapy may be sufficient for short-term tumor control.

For patients who cannot tolerate surgical intervention, radiosurgery can be an alternative. Gerszten and colleagues[50] demonstrated the safety profile and positive clinical outcomes of radiosurgery in a series of 10 spinal meningiomas, as well as other benign spinal tumors; however, it is not common practice and requires further investigation.[51] In cases without open surgery and tissue diagnosis, the treatment is based on radiologic characteristics rather than histopathological confirmation. In addition, if a patient deteriorates neurologically, then surgery may become necessary. Therefore, radiosurgery may be reserved for elderly patients who cannot tolerate surgery or patients with recurrent tumors without spinal cord compression who are not surgical candidates.

SUMMARY/DISCUSSION

Spinal meningiomas represent the most common spinal tumors encountered in adults. Surgical resection is the primary treatment and may afford significant improvement and recovery of neurologic function. Radiation therapy may be used an adjuvant for subtotal resections and higher-grade lesions (WHO grade II or III). Future endeavors in molecular and genetic profiling may guide adjuvant treatment in those with recurrence or higher-grade lesions.

SUPPLEMENTARY DATA

Supplementary data related to this article can be found online at http://dx.doi.org/10.1016/j.nec.2015.11.010.

REFERENCES

1. Mulholland RC. Sir William Gowers 1845-1915. Spine (Phila Pa 1976) 1996;21(9):1106–10.
2. Ostrom QT, Gittleman H, Liao P, et al. CBTRUS statistical report: primary brain and central nervous system tumors diagnosed in the United States in 2007-2011. Neuro Oncol 2014;16(Suppl 4):iv1–63.
3. Albanese V, Platania N. Spinal intradural extramedullary tumors. Personal experience. J Neurosurg Sci 2002;46(1):18–24.
4. Helseth A, Mork SJ. Primary intraspinal neoplasms in Norway, 1955 to 1986. A population-based survey of 467 patients. J Neurosurg 1989;71(5):842–5.
5. Solero CL, Fornari M, Giombini S, et al. Spinal meningiomas: review of 174 operated cases. Neurosurgery 1989;25(2):153–60.
6. Levy WJ Jr, Bay J, Dohn D. Spinal cord meningioma. J Neurosurg 1982;57(6):804–12.
7. Sandalcioglu IE, Hunold A, Muller O, et al. Spinal meningiomas: critical review of 131 surgically treated patients. Eur Spine J 2008;17(8):1035–41.
8. Gottfried ON, Gluf W, Quinones-Hinojosa A, et al. Spinal meningiomas: surgical management and outcome. Neurosurg Focus 2003;14(6):e2.
9. Parisi J, Mena H. Nonglial tumors. In: Nelson J, Parisi J, Schochet S Jr, editors. Principles and practice of neuropathology. St Louis (MO): Mosby; 1993. p. 203–66.
10. Setzer M, Vatter H, Marquardt G, et al. Management of spinal meningiomas: surgical results and a review of the literature. Neurosurg Focus 2007;23(4):E14.
11. Maiuri F, De Caro ML, de Divitiis O, et al. Spinal meningiomas: age-related features. Clin Neurol Neurosurg 2011;113(1):34–8.
12. Schaller B. Spinal meningioma: relationship between histological subtypes and surgical outcome? J Neurooncol 2005;75(2):157–61.
13. Gezen F, Kahraman S, Canakci Z, et al. Review of 36 cases of spinal cord meningioma. Spine (Phila Pa 1976) 2000;25(6):727–31.
14. King AT, Sharr MM, Gullan RW, et al. Spinal meningiomas: a 20-year review. Br J Neurosurg 1998;12(6):521–6.
15. Roux FX, Nataf F, Pinaudeau M, et al. Intraspinal meningiomas: review of 54 cases with discussion of poor prognosis factors and modern therapeutic

management. Surg Neurol 1996;46(5):458–63 [discussion: 463–4].

16. McCormick PC, Torres R, Post KD, et al. Intramedullary ependymoma of the spinal cord. J Neurosurg 1990;72(4):523–32.

17. Sun SQ, Cai C, Ravindra VM, et al. Simpson grade I-III resection of spinal atypical (World Health Organization grade II) meningiomas is associated with symptom resolution and low recurrence. Neurosurgery 2015;76(6):739–46.

18. Klekamp J, Samii M. Surgical results for spinal meningiomas. Surg Neurol 1999;52(6):552–62.

19. Namer IJ, Pamir MN, Benli K, et al. Spinal meningiomas. Neurochirurgia (Stuttg) 1987;30(1):11–5.

20. Peker S, Cerci A, Ozgen S, et al. Spinal meningiomas: evaluation of 41 patients. J Neurosurg Sci 2005;49(1):7–11.

21. Arslantas A, Artan S, Oner U, et al. Detection of chromosomal imbalances in spinal meningiomas by comparative genomic hybridization. Neurol Med Chir (Tokyo) 2003;43(1):12–8 [discussion: 19].

22. Sayagues JM, Tabernero MD, Maillo A, et al. Microarray-based analysis of spinal versus intracranial meningiomas: different clinical, biological, and genetic characteristics associated with distinct patterns of gene expression. J Neuropathol Exp Neurol 2006;65(5):445–54.

23. Ketter R, Henn W, Niedermayer I, et al. Predictive value of progression-associated chromosomal aberrations for the prognosis of meningiomas: a retrospective study of 198 cases. J Neurosurg 2001; 95(4):601–7.

24. Barresi V, Alafaci C, Caffo M, et al. Clinicopathological characteristics, hormone receptor status and matrix metallo-proteinase-9 (MMP-9) immunohistochemical expression in spinal meningiomas. Pathol Res Pract 2012;208(6):350–5.

25. Smith MJ, O'Sullivan J, Bhaskar SS, et al. Loss-of-function mutations in SMARCE1 cause an inherited disorder of multiple spinal meningiomas. Nat Genet 2013;45(3):295–8.

26. Pham MH, Zada G, Mosich GM, et al. Molecular genetics of meningiomas: a systematic review of the current literature and potential basis for future treatment paradigms. Neurosurg Focus 2011;30(5):E7.

27. Karsy M, Guan J, Sivakumar W, et al. The genetic basis of intradural spinal tumors and its impact on clinical treatment. Neurosurg Focus 2015; 39(2):E3.

28. Cohen-Gadol AA, Zikel OM, Koch CA, et al. Spinal meningiomas in patients younger than 50 years of age: a 21-year experience. J Neurosurg 2003;98(3 Suppl):258–63.

29. Tredway TL, Santiago P, Hrubes MR, et al. Minimally invasive resection of intradural-extramedullary spinal neoplasms. Neurosurgery 2006;58(1 Suppl): ONS52–8 [discussion: ONS52–58].

30. Binning MJ, Schmidt MH. Percutaneous placement of radiopaque markers at the pedicle of interest for preoperative localization of thoracic spine level. Spine (Phila Pa 1976) 2010;35(19):1821–5.

31. Amin B, Abdulhak M. Lateral extracavitary approach. In: Baaj A, Mummaneni P, Uribe J, et al, editors. Handbook of spine surgery. New York: Thieme; 2012. p. 290–5.

32. Wiggins GC, Mirza S, Bellabarba C, et al. Perioperative complications with costotransversectomy and anterior approaches to thoracic and thoracolumbar tumors. Neurosurg Focus 2001;11(6):e4.

33. Misra SN, Morgan HW. Avoidance of structural pitfalls in spinal meningioma resection. Neurosurg Focus 2003;14(6):e1.

34. Herman JM, Sonntag VK. Cervical corpectomy and plate fixation for postlaminectomy kyphosis. J Neurosurg 1994;80(6):963–70.

35. Inoue A, Ikata T, Katoh S. Spinal deformity following surgery for spinal cord tumors and tumorous lesions: analysis based on an assessment of the spinal functional curve. Spinal Cord 1996;34(9):536–42.

36. Papagelopoulos PJ, Peterson HA, Ebersold MJ, et al. Spinal column deformity and instability after lumbar or thoracolumbar laminectomy for intraspinal tumors in children and young adults. Spine (Phila Pa 1976) 1997;22(4):442–51.

37. Oxland TR, Lin RM, Panjabi MM. Three-dimensional mechanical properties of the thoracolumbar junction. J Orthop Res Jul 1992;10(4):573–80.

38. Schlenk RP, Kowalski RJ, Benzel EC. Biomechanics of spinal deformity. Neurosurg Focus 2003;14(1):e2.

39. Karikari IO, Nimjee SM, Hodges TR, et al. Impact of tumor histology on resectability and neurological outcome in primary intramedullary spinal cord tumors: a single-center experience with 102 patients. Neurosurgery 2011;68(1):188–97 [discussion: 197].

40. Mimatsu K, Kawakami N, Kato F, et al. Intraoperative ultrasonography of extramedullary spinal tumours. Neuroradiology 1992;34(5):440–3.

41. Simpson D. The recurrence of intracranial meningiomas after surgical treatment. J Neurol Neurosurg Psychiatry 1957;20(1):22–39.

42. Burke D, Hicks R, Stephen J, et al. Assessment of corticospinal and somatosensory conduction simultaneously during scoliosis surgery. Electroencephalogr Clin Neurophysiol 1992;85(6):388–96.

43. Kalkman CJ, Drummond JC, Kennelly NA, et al. Intraoperative monitoring of tibialis anterior muscle motor evoked responses to transcranial electrical stimulation during partial neuromuscular blockade. Anesth Analg 1992;75(4):584–9.

44. Stecker MM. A review of intraoperative monitoring for spinal surgery. Surg Neurol Int 2012;3(Suppl 3): S174–87.

45. Nash CL Jr, Lorig RA, Schatzinger LA, et al. Spinal cord monitoring during operative treatment of the spine. Clin Orthop Relat Res 1977;(126): 100–5.

46. Frankel HL, Hancock DO, Hyslop G, et al. The value of postural reduction in the initial management of closed injuries of the spine with paraplegia and tetraplegia. I. Paraplegia 1969;7(3):179–92.

47. Moazzam AA, Wagle N, Zada G. Recent developments in chemotherapy for meningiomas: a review. Neurosurg Focus 2013;35(6):E18.

48. Sun SQ, Cai C, Murphy RK, et al. Management of atypical cranial meningiomas, part 2: predictors of progression and the role of adjuvant radiation after subtotal resection. Neurosurgery 2014;75(4):356–63 [discussion: 363].

49. Lee KD, DePowell JJ, Air EL, et al. Atypical meningiomas: is postoperative radiotherapy indicated? Neurosurg Focus 2013;35(6):E15.

50. Gerszten PC, Chen S, Quader M, et al. Radiosurgery for benign tumors of the spine using the Synergy S with cone-beam computed tomography image guidance. J Neurosurg 2012;117(Suppl): 197–202.

51. Gerszten PC, Quader M, Novotny J Jr, et al. Radiosurgery for benign tumors of the spine: clinical experience and current trends. Technol Cancer Res Treat 2012;11(2):133–9.

Endoscopic Endonasal and Keyhole Surgery for the Management of Skull Base Meningiomas

Joshua W. Lucas, MD[a], Gabriel Zada, MD, MS[b],*

KEYWORDS

- Endoscopic surgery • Keyhole • Skull base meningiomas

KEY POINTS

- The supraorbital keyhole approach and the endoscopic endonasal approach to the anterior skull base allow for minimally invasive resection of anterior cranial fossa meningiomas.
- The supraorbital keyhole approach has been shown to provide higher rates of gross-total resection of anterior cranial fossa meningiomas when compared with endoscopic techniques.
- Rates of postoperative visual deterioration are higher with the supraorbital keyhole approach when compared with endoscopic techniques.
- The endoscopic endonasal approach has higher rates of postoperative cerebrospinal fluid leakage.
- The individual radiographic and anatomic characteristics of each tumor must be the main determinant in choice of surgical approach.

INTRODUCTION

Anterior skull base meningiomas comprise a diverse group of tumors that can involve a wide range of locations, including the olfactory groove, planum sphenoidale, tuberculum sellae, parasellar region, anterior clinoid process, and petrous ridge.[1] Collectively, these neoplasms account for approximately 10% of all intracranial meningiomas.[2–4] Patients typically present with vision loss and headache, although more uncommon symptoms, such as endocrine disturbances, hydrocephalus, anosmia, or extraocular movement palsies, may occasionally be seen.[5]

Historically, the traditional approaches for the resection of anterior skull base meningiomas have focused on several different transcranial routes, including the more common pterional craniotomy, the unilateral subfrontal craniotomy, and the bilateral subfrontal craniotomy.[6] More recently, introduction of the surgical endoscope into the neurosurgical armamentarium has allowed for minimally invasive approaches to the anterior skull base. The supraorbital keyhole approach and the endoscopic endonasal approach, both techniques in which the endoscope aids immensely in intraoperative visualization, have been developed to provide alternative, less-invasive approaches to aid the resection of these tumors. The determination of which approach is most appropriate depends greatly on the anatomic and imaging features of the meningioma in question and its relationship to critical neurovascular structures[3,7,8] (**Figs. 1** and **2**). In this article, we review the supraorbital keyhole and extended endoscopic endonasal approaches for the resection of anterior skull base meningiomas.

THE SUPRAORBITAL KEYHOLE APPROACH

The supraorbital keyhole approach is a minimally invasive technique that provides access to a

[a] Department of Neurosurgery, Keck School of Medicine at USC, Suite 3300, Los Angeles, CA 90033, USA;
[b] Neuro-Oncology and Endoscopic Pituitary/Skull Base Program, USC Pituitary Center, USC Radiosurgery Center, Keck School of Medicine of USC, Los Angeles, CA, USA
* Corresponding author.
E-mail address: gzada@usc.edu

Neurosurg Clin N Am 27 (2016) 207–214
http://dx.doi.org/10.1016/j.nec.2015.11.008
1042-3680/16/$ – see front matter © 2016 Elsevier Inc. All rights reserved.

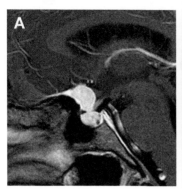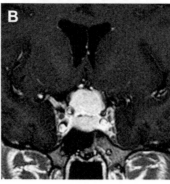

Fig. 1. Sagittal (*A*) and coronal (*B*) MRIs of a typical tuberculum sellae meningioma.

wide range of pathology along the anterior cranial fossa floor and the parasellar region. The addition of endoscopy allows for improved illumination and enhanced visualization of previously hidden areas while still maintaining the benefits of a traditional craniotomy and the familiarity of standard microsurgical dissection techniques. Initial tumor exposure and resection are typically performed with the operative microscope. The endoscope may then be used to magnify the field of view and visualize areas not within the line of sight of the microscope (eg, looking around anatomic corners using angled lenses). Many surgeons advocate for early introduction of the endoscope into the operation to improve visualization of tumor not well visualized using the operative microscope.[9]

The supraorbital keyhole approach is advantageous in its allowance for direct visualization and dissection of tumor from critical neurovascular structures of the anterior skull base. It is truly a minimally invasive approach in that the bone flap typically required is only 3 × 2 cm, and the incision can be made via an eyebrow. It allows the surgeon familiarity of working with standard microneurosurgical instruments during tumor resection, from a standpoint of working between both optic nerves and with an option of working both inferior and superior to the optic chiasm. Additionally, the

supraorbital route does not confine the surgeon to working between confined anatomic triangles to reach the suprasellar region, such as the optico-carotid triangle. Meningiomas that extend superior and lateral to the optic nerve, difficult to reach from a transnasal approach, can be easily removed from the supraorbital route.[10] Compared with pterional and subfrontal craniotomies, this approach requires far less brain retraction to visualize the tumor, and does not necessitate splitting of the Sylvian fissure. Also, unlike transnasal approaches, the supraorbital route has a minimal risk of postoperative cerebrospinal fluid (CSF) leakage.[11] Patients who undergo this procedure have the potential for shorter operative times and hospital stays, improved postoperative pain, and better cosmetic outcomes compared with traditional transcranial approaches.[9] With the addition of endoscopy, better operative field illumination and the ability to achieve an angled view of hidden areas are possible.

Drawbacks of the supraorbital approach include the potential for decreased maneuverability through the small craniotomy, the possibility for damage to the frontotemporal branch of the facial nerve, and the risk of entering the frontal sinus during the bony opening.[6,12] Tumors that extend into the midline depression of the anterior cranial base

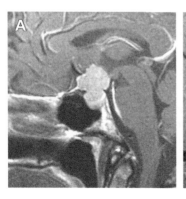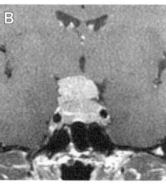

Fig. 2. Sagittal (*A*) and coronal (*B*) MRIs of a typical diaphragm sellae meningioma.

may prove very difficult to resect without the use of angled endoscopes and instruments.[9,11] Similarly, difficulty arises in resection of meningiomas that lie below the line of sight along the frontal floor, such as lesion of the sella and lesions with extension below the sphenoid ridge.[13] Finally, there is a relative blind spot behind the ipsilateral optic nerve from which dissection of firm or adherent meningiomas may prove difficult.

The Supraorbital Keyhole Approach Technique

The keyhole approach uses a trajectory along the anterior cranial fossa floor to access a wide spectrum of pathology. Tailoring the head positioning to the pathology involved in each individual case is critical to the success of the surgery.[9,11–13] The head should be placed in approximately 20° of extension to enable the frontal lobes to fall away from the anterior cranial fossa floor with gravity. Ipsilateral lesions require 15° to 30° of head rotation toward the contralateral side, whereas more midline and contralateral lesions require 45° to 60° of rotation. Stereotactic navigation guidance is often useful for plotting the approach trajectory and avoiding the frontal sinus. In patients with large frontal sinuses, the surgeon must be prepared to cranialize the sinus in the case of accidental entry or avoid it using a more lateral trajectory.

The supraorbital notch is palpated and marks the medial border of the skin incision. The incision is carried through the eyebrow to the lateral eyebrow margin. In rare cases, it may be necessary to extend the incision past the lateral eyebrow margin in a skin crease. The supraorbital nerve should be preserved to prevent permanent numbness of the forehead. The scalp then can be retracted superiorly and the frontalis muscle cut in the line of the incision. A pericranial flap may be elevated at this point and retracted inferiorly along the supraorbital rim, but is not always necessary if the frontal sinus can be avoided.

The anatomic keyhole is subsequently exposed by incising the temporalis fascia. A small burhole is placed at the keyhole using a 4-mm or 5-mm drill bit, and the dura is dissected off the inner table of the skull to facilitate the craniotomy. A small (3 × 2 cm) craniotomy is often sufficient in providing access to address most pathology. Stereotactic navigation can be used to confirm the frontal sinus will not be entered at the medial border of the craniotomy. Also, the proposed trajectory may be confirmed with the navigation system. In cases with extensive superior tumor extension, the orbital rim can be removed with the frontal craniotomy. The inferior extent of the

craniotomy should be as low as possible along the orbital rim to enhance visualization along the anterior cranial fossa floor. The dura is subsequently elevated and any bony protuberances along the anterior cranial base should be flattened with a coarse diamond drill. Additionally, the inner cortex of the frontal bone should be drilled to improve the working angle and aid in visualization.

Attention is subsequently turned to the dura, which is opened and reflected inferiorly (**Fig. 3**). The operating microscope is brought into the field, and the olfactory tract is readily identified and can be followed posteriorly to the optic nerve and opticocarotid cistern. A retractor can be used to elevate the frontal lobe, but is not always required. The proximal Sylvian fissure, along with the prechiasmatic, opticocarotid, and carotidoculomotor cisterns, are widely opened with sharp dissection, and cerebrospinal fluid is patiently suctioned out to relax the frontal lobe (**Fig. 4**). Gravity also will aid in frontal lobe retraction, as arachnoid adhesions are dissected at the base of the frontal lobe and in the Sylvian fissure. The meningioma is identified and its capsule can be opened to permit internal debulking; the tumor is then dissected free from surrounding brain and neurovascular structures using a combination of blunt and sharp dissection.

In the greatest number of cases, most of the microsurgical dissection and tumor removal will be accomplished under the operating microscope. The endoscope is a useful adjunct for both confirmation of removal of the entirety of the tumor or for additional tumor dissection and resection in difficult to visualize areas. A 30° rigid endoscope best serves the purpose of looking around neurovascular structures to assess for residual tumor. Angled endoscopic instrumentation is usually required for further tumor resection under endoscopic guidance. One must use care to

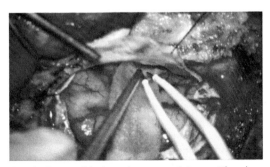

Fig. 3. Supraorbital eyebrow craniotomy. The dura has been opened and reflected inferiorly with retention sutures. A cottonoid is placed on the frontal lobe, and the route of exposure follows the anterior cranial fossa floor back to the optic chiasm.

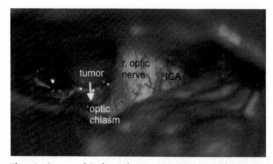

Fig. 4. Supraorbital eyebrow craniotomy. The optic chiasm nerves and chiasm are visualized. The meningioma can often be seen between the optic nerves. The internal carotid artery (ICA) is also visualized lateral to the optic nerves.

avoid collision of the endoscope with proximal structures on entry and removal of the scope, and any thermal injury from the endoscope light. Frequent irrigation and reduction of the magnitude of the light intensity may help prevent the latter issue.

THE ENDOSCOPIC ENDONASAL APPROACH

The endoscopic endonasal approach to meningiomas of the anterior cranial fossa provides a novel alternative to transcranial approaches, allowing for resection of midline tumors extending from the crista galli to the sellar and clival region. The approach is limited laterally by the medial orbital walls anteriorly and the medial opticocarotid recesses posteriorly.[14] The improved illumination and visualization provided by the endoscope enables resection of tumor previously inaccessible by microscopic techniques alone using a minimally invasive route.

Advantages of the endoscopic endonasal approach essentially arise from the ability to achieve important surgical goals early in the operation, before prolonged manipulation of the tumor and critical neurovascular structures. The endonasal route allows for early exposure of the tumor base and subsequent early tumor devascularization.[6,14] Additionally, the optic apparatus, which is often severely compromised by chronic tumor compression, is decompressed early in the procedure without direct manipulation.[15] Other potential advantages include the ability to stay within an intact arachnoid plane during tumor resection, avoiding damage to subchiasmatic perforating vessels and the optic chiasm itself.[6,15] This approach also provides direct exposure of the inferiomedial aspect of the optic canals, allowing for quick decompression of tumor extension to that region, where residual tumor is frequently

left behind using open approaches.[3] Finally, because bone and dura are removed by definition, these approaches may result in more complete (Grade 1) resections, as based on the Simpson grading system.[16] Also, the endoscopic endonasal technique requires no brain retraction, is more cosmetically pleasing, and can often be performed more readily in older patients who are poor surgical candidates.[10]

The major disadvantage of the endoscopic endonasal approach is the difficulty in preventing postoperative CSF leakage.[10,12] A recent meta-analysis of transsphenoidal approaches for tuberculum sellae meningiomas revealed a 20% rate of postoperative CSF leakage.[3] The more anteriorly the bony resection is extended past the tuberculum sellae, the more likely a CSF fistula becomes.[10] Other drawbacks include the lack of 3-dimensional vision and the inability to use traditional microneurosurgical instruments (eg, bipolar cautery forceps) during resection of the meningioma.[6]

The endoscopic endonasal approach is not recommended for lesions larger than 3 cm because of the difficulty in removing tumor superior to the optic nerves, superiorly within the optic canals, and lateral to the anterior clinoid processes and supraclinoid carotid arteries.[6,10,12] Tumors with an eccentric shape, encasement of the carotid arteries and/or anterior communicating artery complex, or involvement of the cavernous sinus may also prove very difficult to resect via an endoscopic endonasal approach.[14,17] Also, the presence of brain edema on preoperative imaging may suggest violation of the arachnoid plane by the tumor, conferring a high risk of postoperative CSF leakage on this approach.[18]

The Endoscopic Endonasal Approach Technique

The standard endoscopic endonasal approach allows access to midline pathology of the sellar and parasellar region.[14,17,19–21] Extended techniques also have been developed that make possible operative corridors from the crista galli to the craniovertebral junction, providing routes by which meningiomas of the anterior cranial base may be resected. In contrast to transcranial approaches, extended endonasal transsphenoidal approaches allow the surgeon to avoid brain retraction, access arterial feeders early in the procedure, and decompress the optic canals before extensive tumor manipulation.

The patient is positioned supine with the head extended and turned toward the surgeon. Stereotactic navigation guidance is used to visualize the extent of bone resection necessary for complete tumor exposure and also for avoidance of critical neurovascular structures. A lumbar drain may be inserted before the operation. A rigid straight 0° endoscope is used for the exposure, which is performed in the usual fashion. In some cases, unilateral middle turbinectomy allows for better working angles in further stages of the operation. If a vascularized nasoseptal flap is to be used for cranial base repair at the end of the procedure, it should be prepared at the onset of the operation. The keel of the sphenoid is removed and a wide anterior sphenoidotomy is performed to maximize visualization and working space, and to minimize collisions of instruments with each other and with the endoscope.

After removal of the sphenoid mucosa, important landmarks of the posterior sphenoid wall, such as the clivus, sella, optic nerve protuberances, opticocarotid recesses, and internal carotid artery protuberances, must be identified to aid in intraoperative orientation. The location of these structures can be confirmed using stereotactic navigation. The navigation system also should be used to identify the margins of the meningioma to assess the amount of bone resection to be performed.

The amount of bony resection must be tailored to an individual's pathology. Tuberculum sellae meningiomas can usually be addressed via a transtuberculum/transplanum approach. The sellar floor is opened with a high-speed drill or ultrasonic bone curette, and a Kerrison rongeur is used to extend the bony opening superiorly (**Fig. 5**). The intercavernous sinus is oftentimes compressed by tumor and usually does not cause significant bleeding, but may be cauterized using a bipolar instrument and cut with endoscopic microscissors. The Kerrison is then used to continue bony removal superiorly past the planum sphenoidale to the falciform ligament and the posterior ethmoidal arteries. The medial optic strut and middle clinoid process must be removed to access the opticocarotid recess during the intradural portion of the procedure without risking perforator injury. The dura can then be opened sharply along the

midline following localization with the neuronavigation instrument and a Doppler flow probe.

Olfactory groove meningiomas must be approached with an extended transcribriform technique (**Fig. 6**). Stereotactic navigation is essential in defining the borders of bone removal. After an anterior sphenoidotomy and wide ethmoid exposure, bone resection is continued rostrally through the ethmoid sinuses to the anterior tumor margin. The bulla ethmoidalis and the ethmoid cells are opened, providing access to the medial orbital wall (lamina papyracea) laterally, the anterior cranial floor superiorly, and the midline septum. The anterior and posterior ethmoidal arteries often provide vascular supply to the tumor and should be coagulated and cut. The posterior limit of the bony exposure is the anterior planum sphenoidale at the level of the posterior ethmoidal arteries.

After confirmation of adequate bony removal with stereotactic navigation, attention can be turned toward tumor resection. The dural base of the tumor should be coagulated and devascularized. The dura can then be opened sharply, taking care not to extend beyond the margins of the tumor initially to prevent herniation of normal brain that will obscure tumor visualization. The tumor is internally debulked to create space for working around the tumor capsule. Early internal decompression takes pressure off of the optic nerves in the first stages of the resection, allowing for tumor mobilization without manipulation of the nerves. Sharp extracapsular dissection should be performed whenever possible using standard microsurgical principles. The anterior tumor border is dissected first, as this is the least likely to involve critical neurovascular structures. The arachnoid covering of the tumor aids in protecting neurovascular structures that may be adherent to the tumor, including the anterior cerebral arteries, superior hypophyseal arteries, infundibulum, and optic nerves. The anterior tumor capsule can be followed superiorly to reach the optic chiasm and nerves, which should be visualized to allow sharp dissection of the tumor capsule from these structures following tumor debulking. Small perforating

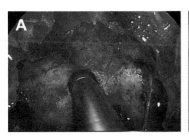
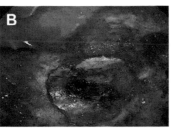

Fig. 5. Endoscopic transsphenoidal approach. (*A*) Drilling of the tuberculum sellae in the approach to the meningioma. (*B*) The completed bony exposure to the dura underlying the tumor.

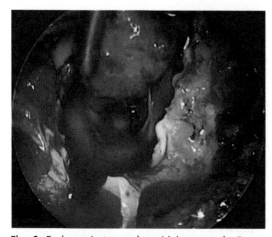

Fig. 6. Endoscopic transsphenoidal approach. Resection of the anterior cranial base meningioma.

arteries to the optic nerves and chiasm (such as the superior hypophyseal artery) should be mobilized and spared when possible. The use of bipolar electrocautery should generally be limited when working in close proximity to optic pathway structures. The tumor can be removed piecemeal or en bloc when freed from surrounding structures.

After complete tumor resection, the resection cavity is thoroughly irrigated and can be inspected with angled (30° or 45°) endoscopes for residual tumor. The anterior cranial floor defect is subsequently closed in a multilayer fashion, often using autologous fascia or fat. A vascularized nasoseptal flap is used for most meningioma cases, and temporary lumbar drainage may be used for 2 to 3 days after the operation to improve the success of the repair (**Fig. 7**).

DISCUSSION

Anterior cranial fossa meningiomas represent a very diverse group of tumors. The most suitable approach for each particular patient therefore largely depends on the intrinsic features of the tumor itself and its anatomic relationships with critical neurovascular structures. The ultimate goal of meningioma surgery is maximal tumor resection and adequate decompression of critical

neurovascular structures with minimal morbidity, and the choice of approach should always reflect that goal.

Meningioma location is arguably the most important variable, as some tumor locations are much more amenable to the endoscopic endonasal approach, such as meningiomas of the planum sphenoidale or olfactory groove. Anterior clinoid tumors and lesions of the diaphragma sellae are usually more suited for traditional transcranial approaches. Meningiomas of the tuberculum sellae may be treated via either approach. Tumors that involve the lateral optic canal are more suitably treated via a transcranial approach, as the endoscopic endonasal technique does not provide sufficient access to this area.[6] In general, smaller tumors of the midline are considered good candidates for endoscopic endonasal procedures.

Tumor size is another important characteristic in the determination of optimal surgical approach. According to Fahlbusch and Schott[22] and Raco and colleagues,[23] the size of the tumor influences visual outcome, with patients harboring tumors smaller than 3 cm having better visual outcomes than those with tumors larger than 3 cm. Transcranial approaches are almost universally used for tumors larger than 3 cm, as these tumors inherently extend laterally to areas inaccessible from an endonasal approach, and often encase critical neurovascular structures that require microsurgical dissection with standard neurosurgical instruments. Larger meningiomas (>3 cm in diameter) located more anteriorly along the skull base in the region of the olfactory groove and planum sphenoidale have been successfully removed using extended endoscopic endonasal approaches as long as lateral extension remains limited.

The endoscopic endonasal approach has been shown to result in shorter hospital stays, shorter operative times, and less blood loss when compared with transcranial procedures.[8] Other studies also have shown decreased hemorrhagic complications, decreased frequency of injuries to the brain parenchyma, and fewer seizures with the endoscopic endonasal route.[3] Potentially the

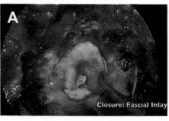
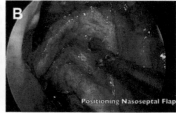

Fig. 7. Endoscopic transsphenoidal approach. (*A*) Placement of a fascial inlay underneath the bone edges. (*B*) Placement of a pedicled nasoseptal flap for the prevention of postoperative CSF leakage.

largest advantage of this approach, however, is improved visual outcomes when compared with transcranial procedures. The endoscopic endonasal technique theoretically allows for reduced manipulation of the chronically compressed optic chiasm, and improved visualization and preservation of perforating vessels to the optic chiasm. The biggest drawback of the endoscopic endonasal technique is the risk of CSF leakage postoperatively, rates of which in several series range from 23% to 40%.[1,6,14] Vascularized, pedicled nasoseptal flaps have been shown to be the most effective means of cranial base reconstruction for these large osteodural defects, and prophylactic harvest and placement of these flaps in select cases has improved CSF leakage rates.[24,25] With time, experienced centers have shown improvements in the rates of postoperative CSF leaks ranging between 5% and 10%.

Traditional transcranial approaches, such as the pterional craniotomy and unilateral or bilateral subfrontal craniotomy, have been shown to have very high rates of gross-total resection in anterior cranial fossa meningiomas, and should still be reserved as good options for large or highly complex meningiomas. In a recent literature review by Gadgil and colleagues,[6] 85% of 993 transcranial procedures for anterior cranial fossa meningiomas were defined as Simpson Grade I or II resections. The most common reason for incomplete resection was tumor surrounding the internal carotid arteries or the anterior communicating artery complex. These approaches, however, carry a higher risk of worsened vision postoperatively, as compared with the endoscopic endonasal approach; as much as 13% to 20% in some large literature reviews,[1,6,14] although the potential for selection bias in choosing an approach based on anatomic tumor features may exist. Alternatively, this could possibly be due to the difficulty in visualizing subchiasmatic perforators via these approaches as compared with an endoscopic endonasal approach. Transcranial approaches also have been associated with temporalis muscle atrophy, mandibular pain, alopecia, and numbness around the incision site.[9]

The supraorbital keyhole approach allows for a familiar approach through a craniotomy large enough to perform bimanual microdissection using standard neurosurgical instruments, avoidance of sinonasal morbidity associated with the endonasal approach, and the ability to use the endoscope concurrently to ensure complete resection.[11] Several large recent series of patients treated solely with the supraorbital keyhole approach have demonstrated results similar to traditional transcranial approaches, with gross-total resection seen in more than 80% of patients and worsening of visual field deficit in fewer than 20% of patients.[9,26]

Recent comparative meta-analyses have shown that endoscopic endonasal procedures are associated with significantly higher rates of postoperative improvement in vision compared with transcranial approaches.[3,15] One analysis showed improvement in vision in 60% of transcranial patients as compared with 74% of endoscopic endonasal patients.[3] These studies also show significantly higher rates of gross-total resection with transcranial procedures.[27] Again, it is important to note that selection bias may contribute to these results, as more favorable patients with smaller, midline tumors are oftentimes favored for endoscopic resections instead of transcranial approaches.[6,14]

Future improvements and refinements of surgical techniques could alter the decision-making process for anterior cranial fossa meningiomas. Improvements in endoscopic instrumentation could enable future surgeons to emulate traditional microneurosurgical dissection techniques and increase rates of gross-total resections. Also, more widespread use of vascularized, pedicled nasoseptal flaps could decrease the rates of postoperative CSF leakage. Some centers are even combining techniques, with a combination of a supraorbital keyhole approach and an endoscopic endonasal transsphenoidal approach, performed either in a 2-stage operation or in a single-stage with 2 surgeons.[28]

SUMMARY

The endoscopic endonasal approach and supraorbital keyhole approach are both useful minimally invasive techniques for resection of anterior skull base meningiomas. Whereas the endonasal route demonstrates improved postoperative visual function in several studies, the supraorbital technique has shown to be associated with higher rates of gross-total resection. Although risk of postoperative CSF leak from an endoscopic endonasal approach is a major drawback to this route, surgeon experience and the use of pedicled naso-septal flaps have helped reduce these rates substantially. Despite the advantages and disadvantages of each approach, the individual characteristics of each tumor must be the main determinant in choice of surgical approach.

REFERENCES

1. Gardner PA, Kassam AB, Thomas A, et al. Endoscopic endonasal resection of anterior cranial base meningiomas. Neurosurgery 2008;63:36–54.

2. Khan OH, Anand VK, Schwartz TH. Endoscopic endonasal resection of skull base meningiomas: the significance of a "cortical cuff" and brain edema compared with careful case selection and surgical experience in predicting morbidity and extent of resection. Neurosurg Focus 2014;37(4):E7.

3. de Divitiis E, Esposito F, Cappabianca P, et al. Tuberculum sellae meningiomas: high route or low route? A series of 51 consecutive cases. Neurosurgery 2008;62:556–63.

4. Ajlan AM, Choudhri O, Hwang P, et al. Meningiomas of the tuberculum and diaphragm sellae. J Neurol Surg B Skull Base 2015;76:74–9.

5. Wang Q, Lu XJ, Li B, et al. Extended endoscopic endonasal transsphenoidal removal of tuberculum sellae meningiomas: a preliminary report. J Clin Neurosci 2009;16:889–93.

6. Gadgil N, Thomas JG, Takashima M, et al. Endoscopic resection of tuberculum sellae meningiomas. J Neurol Surg B Skull Base 2013;74:201–10.

7. Fatemi N, Dusick JR, de Paiva Neto MA, et al. Endonasal versus supra-orbital keyhole removal of craniopharyngiomas and tuberculum sellae meningiomas. Neurosurgery 2008;62:325–30.

8. Kitano M, Taneda M, Nakao Y. Postoperative improvement in visual function in patients with tuberculum sellae meningiomas: results of the extended transsphenoidal and intracranial approaches. J Neurosurg 2007;107:337–46.

9. Gazzeri R, Nishiyama Y, Teo C. Endoscopic supraorbital eyebrow approach for the surgical treatment of extraaxial and intraaxial tumors. Neurosurg Focus 2014;37(4):E20.

10. Bowers CA, Altay T, Couldwell WT. Surgical decision-making strategies in tuberculum sellae meningioma resection. Neurosurg Focus 2011;30(5):E1.

11. Zada G. Editorial: The endoscopic supraorbital keyhole approach. Neurosurg Focus 2014;37(4):E21.

12. Fatemi N, Dusick J, de Paiva Neto M, et al. Endonasal versus supraorbital keyhole removal of craniopharyngiomas and tuberculum sellae meningiomas. Neurosurgery 2009;64:269–86.

13. Wilson DA, Duong H, Teo C, et al. The supraorbital endoscopic approach for tumors. World Neurosurg 2014;82:S72–80.

14. de Divitiis E, Esposito F, Cappabianca P, et al. Endoscopic transnasal resection of anterior cranial fossa meningiomas. Neurosurg Focus 2008;25(6):E8.

15. Wang Q, Lu XJ, Ji WY, et al. Visual outcome after extended endoscopic endonasal transsphenoidal surgery for tuberculum sellae meningiomas. World Neurosurg 2010;73(6):694–700.

16. Simpson D. The recurrence of intracranial meningiomas after surgical treatment. J Neurol Neurosurg Psychiatry 1957;20:22–39.

17. de Divitiis E, Cavallo LM, Esposito F, et al. Extended endoscopic transsphenoidal approach for tuberculum sellae meningiomas. Neurosurgery 2007;61:229–38.

18. Ganna A, Dehdashti AR, Karabatsou K, et al. Frontobasal interhemispheric approach for tuberculum sellae meningiomas: long term visual outcome. Br J Neurosurg 2009;23:422–30.

19. Ditzel Filho L, Prevadello DM, Jamshidi AO, et al. Endoscopic endonasal approach for removal of tuberculum sellae meningiomas. Neurosurg Clin N Am 2015;26:349–61.

20. Kulwin C, Schwartz TH, Cohen-Gadol AA. Endoscopic extended transsphenoidal resection of tuberculum sellae meningiomas: nuances of neurosurgical technique. Neurosurg Focus 2013;35(6):E6.

21. Liu JK, Hattar E. Anderson Eloy J: Endoscopic endonasal approach for olfactory groove meningiomas: operative technique and nuances. Neurosurg Clin N Am 2015;26:377–88.

22. Fahlbusch R, Schott W. Pterional surgery of meningiomas of the tuberculum sellae and planum sphenoidale: surgical results with special consideration of ophthalmological and endocrinological outcomes. J Neurosurg 2002;96:235–43.

23. Raco A, Bristot R, Domenicucci M, et al. Meningiomas of the tuberculum sellae. Our experience in 69 cases surgically treated between 1973 and 1993. J Neurosurg Sci 1999;43:253–62.

24. Cavallo LM, Messina A, Esposito F, et al. Skull base reconstruction in the extended endoscopic transsphenoidal approach for suprasellar lesions. J Neurosurg 2007;107:713–20.

25. Hadad G, Bassagasteguy L, Carrau RL, et al. A novel reconstructive technique after endoscopic expanded endonasal approaches: vascular pedicle nasoseptal flap. Laryngoscope 2006;116:1882–6.

26. Romani R, Laakso A, Kangasniemi M, et al. Lateral supraorbital approach applied to tuberculum sellae meningiomas: experience with 52 consecutive patients. Neurosurgery 2012;70:1504–19.

27. Komotar RJ, Starke RM, Raper DM, et al. Endoscopic endonasal versus open transcranial resection of anterior midline skull base meningiomas. World Neurosurg 2012;77(5–6):713–24.

28. Van Lindert EJ, Grotenhuis JA. The combined supraorbital keyhole-endoscopic endonasal transsphenoidal approach to sellar, perisellar, and frontal skull base tumors: surgical technique. Minim Invasive Neurosurg 2009;52:281–6.

The Contemporary Role of Stereotactic Radiosurgery in the Treatment of Meningiomas

Or Cohen-Inbar, MD, PhD[a],*, Cheng-chia Lee, MD[b],
Jason P. Sheehan, MD, PhD[a]

KEYWORDS

- Meningioma • Stereotactic radiosurgery • Gamma knife • Cyberknife • Novalis • Trilogy
- Tomotherapy

KEY POINTS

- Stereotactic radiosurgery (SRS) is an important treatment option in the management meningiomas and can be used as upfront or adjuvant treatment modality.
- SRS seems to afford a high and durable rate of tumor control with a very low complication rate and a high safety profile.
- Complications resulting from radiosurgery are relatively rare, and they are typically manageable and temporary.
- For many patients with meningiomas, the risk to benefit ratio profile seems favorable compared with the treatment alternatives of radical resection or tumor progression.
- Multicenter-driven, evidence-based, objective outcome evaluations and international consortium efforts promise to continue improving and advance better patients care.

INTRODUCTION

Meningioma Classification and Epidemiology

Meningiomas are among the most common intracranial tumors in adults.[1] These tumors are thought to originate from the arachnoidal cap cells,[2] forming the outer layer of the arachnoid membrane villi (the latter facilitates cerebrospinal fluid drainage into the dural sinuses and veins). Intracranial meningiomas account for 24% to 33% of primary brain tumors[3] and have an incidence of approximately 6 in 100,000, but they can be discovered incidentally on neuroimaging for other concerns, or at autopsy.[4] In the absence of genetic or environmental risk factors, the incidence of meningiomas increases with age, occurring primarily in the sixth to eighth decades of life.[5,6] Meningiomas are histologically characterized as benign, atypical, or malignant (also known as anaplastic) by the 3-tiered World Health Organization (WHO) classification scheme. Most meningiomas are benign (ie, WHO grade I),[1,7] slow-growing tumors. WHO grade I meningiomas are discussed much more frequently in the literature owing to their high incidence and the long-term patient survival associated with contemporary management strategies.

Disclosures: The authors have no personal or institutional financial interest in drugs or materials in relation to this paper.
[a] Department of Neurological Surgery, University of Virginia Health Sciences Center, Box 800212, Charlottesville, VA 22908, USA; [b] Neurological Institute, Taipei Veteran General Hospital, National Yang-Ming University, 17F., No.201, Sec. 2, Shipai Rd., Beitou District, Taipei 11217, Taiwan
* Corresponding author.
E-mail address: oc2f@virginia.edu

Neurosurg Clin N Am 27 (2016) 215–228
http://dx.doi.org/10.1016/j.nec.2015.11.006
1042-3680/16/$ – see front matter © 2016 Elsevier Inc. All rights reserved.

The WHO scheme has been revised dramatically in recent years, including a major revision in 2000. The latest update from 2007 resulted in the redistribution of many meningiomas into different classes.[8] According to previous classification schemes, approximately 90% of meningiomas were classified as benign, 5% to 7% as atypical, and 3% to 5% as malignant.[9] In the current pathologic classification, approximately 35% of all meningiomas are atypical (WHO grade II) or malignant (WHO grade III).[10] WHO grade II and III meningiomas behave very differently and quite often exhibit an aggressive course accompanied by recurrence, invasion, and even distant metastasis.[2,11] The 5- and 10-year overall survival rates for all meningioma patients are high at 82% and 64%, respectively,[5] but the prognosis for aggressive, higher grade meningiomas is much worse.[12,13] The 5- and 10-year survival rates for patients with aggressive meningiomas are 65% and 51%, respectively.[14] Grades II and III tumors are more likely to recur and are associated with worse overall survival[2,12] (**Tables 1** and **2**).

Brief Overview of Resection

Microsurgical resection has traditionally been regarded as the treatment of choice for meningiomas, still playing a significant role in the management of many patients. Resection offers several advantages, including a histologic confirmation of the tumor features, relief of compression and mass effect imposed on neurovascular structures, and, in the instance of gross total resection, the chance of a cure. Control rates after resection vary depending on the extent of resection; this observation was first described by Simpson in 1957.[15] Simpson reported that after a complete resection (ie, excision of tumor, its dural attachment and any abnormal bone, later defined as Simpson grade I), tumor recurrences at 5, 10, and 15 years are 5%, 10%, and 30%, respectively.[15] Since this landmark report, more recent studies reported a wide range of tumor control, progression-free survival, and recurrence rates, mirroring at least in part the evolving technology and surgical skills. A literature review of major surgical resection series for meningiomas is presented in **Tables 1** and **2**.

Despite tremendous advances in neurosurgical technique and equipment, postoperative morbidity continues to taint open complete removal of many cranial base tumors, with an incidence of temporary and permanent postoperative cranial nerve deficits as high as 44% and 56%, respectively.[16,17] Operative mortality rates in some series was reported to be as high as 9% (median, 3.6%).[16–18] Thus, the advantage of a radical tumor resection must be weighed against the associated surgical morbidity. Subtotal resections may be required for meningiomas that involve major draining veins or cranial nerves. Lesions adjacent to critical neurovascular structures, especially skull base meningiomas, often do not allow for a safe complete resection, which can lead to lower local control and increased risk of tumor progression or recurrence.[19,20] Resection carries the added risk of surgery-related morbidity.[19] In such instances, where a complete resection is not prudent or feasible, a cytoreductive or "near total" resection may be advantageous to relieve mass effect and decrease the remaining target volume for radiosurgery (later termed the adaptive hybrid surgery approach).

The need for a Simpson grade I/II resection has been repeatedly called into question in modern times for patients with WHO grade I meningiomas.[21] Some reports state no significant difference in recurrence-free survival between patients undergoing a Simpson grade I, II, III, or IV resection.[21] Given the option of adjuvant treatment (eg, stereotactic radiosurgery [SRS]) for small residual or recurrent WHO grade I meningiomas, a gross total or near total resection may not be as important to progression-free survival as when Simpson's work was published in 1957.

The Evolution of Radiosurgery

Since its inception more than 60 years ago, SRS techniques and technology have evolved significantly, but its fundamental principles remain unchanged. In 2006, the American College of Radiology and the American Society for Radiation Oncology published practice guidelines for the performance of SRS.[22] A multidisciplinary, collaborative effort among neurosurgeons, radiation oncologists, and medical physicists was recommended to optimize the quality and operational efficiency of successful SRS. A subsequent publication put forth in 2007 by the SRS Task Force (a joint committee of the American Association of Neurologic Surgeons and the Congress of Neurologic Surgeons), in conjunction with the American Society for Radiation Oncology, distinguished between SRS and fractionated stereotactic radiotherapy.[23,24] This same joint task force, further defined SRS to be "typically performed in a single session, using a rigidly attached stereotactic guiding device, other immobilization technology and/or a stereotactic imaging guidance system, but can be performed in a limited number of sessions, up to a maximum of five."

Table 1
Major series of treatment for meningiomas with radiosurgery with long-term follow-up stratified based on location

Location	Author, Year	No. of Patients	Median Tumor Volume (mL)	Median Follow-Up	Patients with >10 y Assessment, n (%)	Actuarial Local Control (%)		Actuarial PFS, n (%)	Morbidity/ Complications (%)
						5 y	10 y		
All	Kondziolka et al,[49] 2014	290	5.5	56	29 (10)	—	87.7	80.3	17.9
	Santacroce et al,[47] 2012	4565	4.8	63	8.4	92.6	82	95.2 (5 y), 88.6 (10 y)	6.6
	Pollock et al,[76] 2012	416	7.3	60	17	96	89	97 (5 y), 94 (10 y)	11
	Zada et al,[77] 2010	116	3.4	75	—	98.9	84	94 (10 y)	8
	Kondziolka et al,[46] 2008	972	7.4 mean	48 mean	7.7	—	91, 95	—	7.7
	Kollova et al,[71] 2007	325	4.4	60	NR	97.9	90	—	5.7
	Dibiase et al,[35] 2004	121	4.5	54	NR	86.2	—	86.2 (5 y)	8.3
	Stafford et al,[78] 2001	168	—	40	NR	93	—	—	13
Convexity	Kondziolka et al,[56] 2009	115	7	31	NR	95.3	—	—	9.6
	Pamir et al,[59] 2007	43	—	46	NR	89	—	—	—
	Kim et al,[79] 2005	26	4.7	33 mean	NR	96	—	—	—
Skull base	Cohen-Inbar et al,[51] 2015	135	4.7	102.5	37	100	88.1	95.4 (10 y)	14.8
	Iwai et al,[29] 2008	108	8.1	86.1	23	—	83	83 (10 y)	6
	Kreil et al,[39] 2005	200	6.5	95	—	98.5	97	97.2 (10 y)	2.5
Parasellar	Williams et al,[80] 2011	138	7.5	76	16	95.4	—	69 (10 y)	10
	Skeie et al,[81] 2010	100	—	82 mean	20	94.2	91.6	—	6
	Hasegawa et al,[82] 2007	115	14	62	9	94	92	73.5 (10 y)	12
	Nicolato et al,[83] 2001	122	8.3	49	—	96.5	—	96.5 (5 y)	4
	Lee et al,[28] 2002	159	6.45 mean	39	—	96.9	93	93.1 (10 y)	6.9
FM	Starke et al,[84] 2010	5	6.8	72	—	80	—	—	0

Abbreviations: FM, foramen magnum; PFS, progression-free survival.
Data from Refs.[28,29,35,39,46,47,49,51,56,59,71,76–84]

Table 2
Literature review of aggressive meningiomas treated by SRS

Author, Year	WHO Grade	Patient Number	Control Rate	PFS	Overall Survival
Ojemann et al,[85] 2000	3	19 (31)	—	26% at 5 y	40% at 5 y
Stafford et al,[78] 2001	2 3	13 9	68% at 5 y 0% at 5 y	—	76% at 5 y[a] 0% at 5 y[a]
Harris et al,[86] 2003	2 3	18 12	—	83% at 5 y 72% at 5 y	59% at 5, 10 y 59% at 5 y, 0% at 10 y
Huffmann et al,[87] 2005	2	15 (21)	93% at 6 mo	—	100% at 35 mo
Kondziolka et al,[46] 2008	2 3	54 29	50% at 2 y 17% at 15 mo	—	—
Attia et al,[88] 2012	2	24	75% at 1 y 51% at 2 y 44% at 5 y	40% at 2 y, 25% at 5 y	92% at 1 y, 67% at 2 y, 52% at 5 y
Mori et al,[89] 2013	2 3	19 (22) 4	74% at 1 y 54% at 2 y 34% at 3 y	—	—
Tamura et al,[90] 2013	2 3	9 7	29% at 40.5 mo	—	—
Ferraro et al,[12] 2014	2 3	31 4	—	95.7% at 1 y, 70.1% at 3 y 0% at 1, 3 y	92.4% at 1 y, 83.4% at 3 y 33% at 1, 3 y

Abbreviations: PFS, progression-free survival; SRS, stereotactic radiosurgery (these series are all gamma-knife radiosurgery based); WHO, World Health Organization.
^a Cause-specific survival.
Data from Refs.[12,46,78,85–90]

The ionizing radiation used in SRS is most commonly either gamma radiation (usually emitted by the radioactive Cobalt [Co] isotope 60) or accelerated electrons from linear accelerators (LINAC). Modern SRS systems include the gamma knife (Elekta AB, Stockholm, Sweden), Cyberknife (Accuray, Sunnyvale, CA), Edge (Varian Medical Systems, Palo Alto, CA), Novalis (Brainlab AG, Feldkirchen, Germany), and Infini (MASEP, City of Industry, CA) to name a few.

THE RADIOBIOLOGY OF RADIOSURGERY

SRS was conceived with the aim of inactivating or lesioning intracranial targets through the intact skull with the use of many highly focused, ionizing beams of radiation using stereotaxis and image guidance. Although each beam itself delivers a very low level of radiation, the target focus at which the beams converge receives a concentrated high dose of radiation. The normal brain surrounding the focus receives a significantly lesser amount of collateral radiation than the target owing to the steep dose fall off. The mathematical analog of radiosurgery would be the step function although radiosurgery simply approaches such a theoretic absolute. The classic 4 *R*s of radiation therapy (ie, the most important biological factors influencing the responses of tumors and normal tissues to fractionated treatment), that is, repair, reassortment, repopulation and reoxygenation, are of lesser importance in radiosurgery than they are in radiation therapy.

The biology of radiosurgery is not entirely understood. In fact, the linear quadratic model is not believed to adequately predict outcomes associated with intracranial SRS.[24] It seems clear that the cellular response differs dramatically when cells are irradiated with doses of greater than 5 Gy at a time, than when irradiated with lower doses, as practiced in conventional radiotherapy.[25] Certainly, radiosurgery induces many of the same single- and double-stranded DNA breaks that fractionated radiation therapy does. SRS has been shown to inflict both direct cytotoxic effect as well as to abrogate tumor angiogenesis by promoting endothelial apoptosis and other vascular changes.[25,26] The dose heterogeneity inherent to multi-isocenteric–based planning in gamma knife radiosurgery platforms, the so called "hot spots" phenomena, has been assigned a possible additional radiobiologic advantage for the treatment of small to moderately sized intracerebral volumes.[27]

Meningiomas are classically considered as a late responding tissue, and as such require a higher biologically effective dose. Radiosurgery can be used to deliver a higher biologically effective dose to a tumor than might be afforded by conventional radiotherapy. Provided that the dose falloff is steep enough to surrounding structures, the higher biologically effective dose should translate to a greater rate of local tumor control while still offering a low rate of complications.[25–27]

RADIOSURGICAL RESULTS FOR WORLD HEALTH ORGANIZATION CLASS I BENIGN MENINGIOMAS

SRS has demonstrated its safety and efficacy in the control of benign meningiomas, particularly for small to moderately sized tumors. Lesions should optimally be less than 3 cm in diameter (approximately 10 cm^3 in volume), have distinct margins, and located at sufficient distance from functionally important brain regions or other radiosensitive structures to permit a safe delivery of an adequate prescription dose to the tumor. SRS has been applied most frequently to patients whose meningioma present significant management challenges.[28–30] These challenges are often related to tumor location, patient age, comorbidities, recurrence after incomplete resection, and risks of neurologic morbidity if resection is pursued. The skull base typically presents many such treatment challenges. Refer to **Table 1** for a review of the literature and to **Figs. 1** and **2** for typical meningioma patients treated with radiosurgery.

The Effect of Dose and Tumor Volume on Prognosis

The margin dose for meningiomas varies, depending on their location, proximity to radiosensitive structures (the optic apparatus, cochlea, or brainstem, for example), and histologic grade. The general ranges of radiosurgical margin doses for WHO grade I, II, and III meningiomas are 12 to 16, 16 to 20, and 18 to 24 Gy, respectively.[31,32] For WHO grade I meningiomas, excellent local control of 90% or greater has consistently been achieved with 12 to 16 Gy.[33] Furthermore, no improvement with marginal doses greater than 15 Gy versus less than 15 Gy was reported.[34]

With respect to tumor size (volume), within the confines of single session SRS (up to 10–12 mL), DiBiase and colleagues[35] reported a 91.9% 5-year disease-free survival rate for patients with meningiomas less than 10 cm^3 as opposed to 68% for larger tumors. Kondziolka and colleagues[34] reported excellent outcomes with SRS for meningiomas up to a diameter of 3.0 cm or a volume of 7.5 cm^3. Other authors have found comparable good local control rates and fewer radiation-related complications associated with treatment of smallest quartile meningiomas (4.8% in lesions <3.2 cm^3), compared with largest quartile meningiomas (22.6% in lesions >9.6 cm^3).[36,37] Pollock and colleagues[36,37] found no difference in the progression-free survival rate at 7 years in patients who underwent either radiosurgery or a Simpson grade 1 resection for meningiomas less than 3.5 cm in diameter.[15,30]

Tumor Control Rates Based on the Duration of Follow-up

Published SRS tumor control rates for WHO grade I meningiomas are high (92%–100%).[28,29,34,38–41] Such tumor control is comparable with that of a complete surgical resection with dura resection (Simpson's grade 1)[15,30] with added benefit of a low toxicity as well.[42–44] These control rates average 91% and 88% at 5 and 10 years, respectively (see **Figs. 1** and **2**).[29,35,45,46] Most reports are based on retrospective cohorts with median follow-up durations of less than 5 years.[28–30,34,35,38,39] Reports having long-term tumor control and neurologic status are limited. **Table 1** lists the major SRS series for WHO grade I meningiomas with long term follow-up stratified based on location. Kondziolka and colleagues[41] reported patient outcomes up to 10 years after radiosurgery and found a tumor control rate of 95%. This figure decreased to 89% at 10 years when including adjacent or new tumor growth away from the primary target as treatment failure (so-called out of field recurrence). Santacroce and colleagues[47] reported an 88.6% tumor progression-free survival at 10 years. Bledsoe and colleagues[48] reported a tumor control rate of 99% at 7 years and a neurologic complication rate of 18% in skull base tumors.

In 8 long-term series (see **Table 1**), the 10-year actuarial rate of tumor control varied from 69% to 92%.[29,30,36,46,47] Fokas and colleagues[44] reported 5-year rates of local control, overall survival, and cause-specific survival to be 92.9%, 88.7%, and 97.2%, respectively. These parameters decreased in 10 years to 87.5%, 74.1%, and 97.2%, respectively. On multivariate analysis, the authors reported tumor location ($P = .029$) and age less than 66 years ($P = .031$) to be predictors of local control and overall survival.[44] Kondziolka

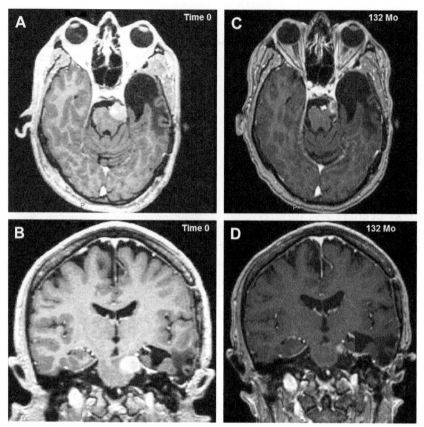

Fig. 1. A 60-year-old male patient treated for a left tentorial petroclival meningioma abutting the midbrain. Treatment volume was 2 mL, given 12 Gy to the 40% isodose line. Karnofsky performance status (KPS) on presentation was 90. (*A*, *B*) Axial and coronal T1-weighted imaging contrast enhanced at the time of gamma knife radiosurgery (time 0), respectively. (*C*, *D*) Axial and coronal T1-weighted imaging contrast enhanced images respectively, taken at 132 months follow-up, presenting the local control. KPS at his last follow-up was 90.

and colleagues[49] reported a series with 53% of patients having residual or recurrent tumors after initial surgical resection and subsequent treatment with SRS. At intervals of 10 or more years after SRS, long-term tumor control rates were sustained.[49]

Stereotactic Radiosurgery as a Primary Treatment Modality

In the modern era, with increasing patient awareness, quality of life and availability of imaging devices and indications, meningiomas are detected by neuroimaging and given the presumptive diagnosis of a meningioma. SRS has been used to treat patients with skull base meningiomas for which there is no firm, histologic diagnosis, rather radiologic findings or progression solely. Spiegelmann and colleagues[50] reported a cohort of imaging-based diagnosed meningiomas treated with SRS. The authors reported a 98% tumor control rate. In a separate cohort of 219 image diagnosed predominantly skull base meningiomas

treated with radiosurgery, the actuarial tumor control rate at 5 years was 93.2% and the actuarial rate of diagnosing a tumor other than a meningioma was 2.3% at 5 years.[38] Most SRS series include lesions for which no tissue diagnosis is available, showing comparable outcome parameters. It seems to be safe to treat a lesion having all the clinical and radiologic features of a benign meningioma, negating the need for tissue diagnosis in these cases. Lesions should be followed as suggested previously and a biopsy/tissue diagnosis should be prompted if these change their clinical or radiologic behavior or appearance in a more ominous fashion.

Long-term Radiosurgical Outcomes

Long-term follow-up of any procedure and for any neoplastic pathology is more likely to uncover late complications and treatment related morbidity. We recently reported a cohort of 135 patients with a WHO grade I skull base meningioma treated with a single-session gamma knife radiosurgery

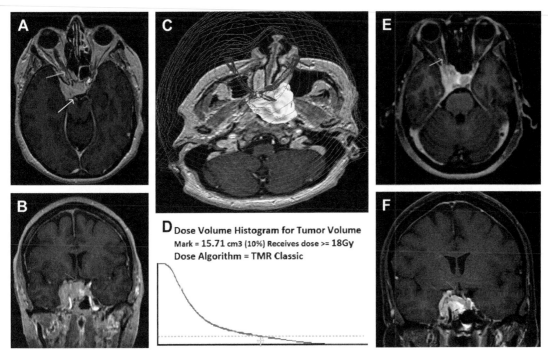

Fig. 2. Parasellar meningioma patient. (*A, B*) Axial and coronal preradiosurgical T1-weighted imaging plus contrast MRI, respectively. A right parasellar and cavernous sinus meningioma is shown. The lesion abuts the right optic nerve and has a wide contrast surface with it (*blue arrow*) and with the optic chiasm (*red arrow*). The right oculomotor nerve (cranial nerve III) is also compressed (*yellow arrow*). The patient was treated with hypofractionated gamma-knife radiosurgery using 5 fractions with 5 Gy per fraction. (*C*) Treatment plan. (*D*) A dose–volume histogram for the treatment is presented. (*E, F*) At 12 months after radiosurgical axial and coronal T1-weighted imaging plus contrast imaging, the tumor has regressed, which is more clearly seen owing to the lack of optic nerve and optic chiasm compression (*blue and red arrows*, respectively).

and a minimum of 60 months of follow-up.[51] The cohort comprised 54.1% males (n = 73). The median age was 54 years (range, 19–80) and median tumor volume was 4.7 cm³ (range, 0.5–23). Median margin dose was 15 Gy (range, 7.5–36). Median follow-up was 102.5 months (range, 60.1–235.4). Tumor control and post-SRS clinical neurologic preservation or improvement (both subjective and objective as quantified by the Karnofsky performance status) was shown to be influenced by the pre-SRS performance status (Karnofsky performance status).[51] Favorable outcome (both tumor control and post-gamma knife radiosurgery clinical neurologic preservation or improvement), a parameter that unifies the clinical and oncologic goals of quality of life and tumor control, was reported in 60.8% of patients (n = 79) at last follow-up.[51]

Reported long-term signs and symptoms included intermittent headache, which was reported as the most common complaint in 34.8%, followed by dizziness (15.6%) and SRS-induced cranial nerve deficit (14.8%). Of the cranial nerves affected, the trigeminal nerve was most affected,

followed by the vestibulocochlear and optic nerves. The prevalence of radiosurgery related cranial nerve deficits is comparable to reports with a shorter follow-up time, ranging from 4.8% to 22.6%.[36,37] Thus, it seems that SRS carries a defined and acceptable risk of cranial neuropathies in proximity of the treatment volume, that may approach as high as 15% over a follow-up period of almost 20 years.

Skull Base Meningiomas

Skull base meningiomas often abut or encase neurovascular structures and may extend into more than 1 cranial fossa. Hence, many skull base meningiomas are an ideal target for radiosurgery given the difficulty with achieving a complete resection. In a similar manner to the evolution of treatment approaches for vestibular schwannomas, SRS has overtaken microsurgery at many centers as the preferred initial treatment modality for the majority of patients with skull base meningiomas less than 3 cm in size.[46,52] SRS may be used as a complimentary approach to microsurgery as well. Comparable results are reported for gamma knife and LINAC-based radiosurgery systems.

Kondziolka and colleagues[46] reported a series of 972 patients with meningiomas in different locations with predominance to the skull base. The 5-, 10-, and 15-year tumor control rates were 93%, 87%, and 87%, respectively. These local tumor control rates were achieved with a median dose of 13 Gy to the tumor margin.[46] In a previous series of patients with cavernous sinus meningiomas, the same group reported 5- and 10-year local tumor control rates of 93%.[28] In another series of 200 patients with skull base meningiomas treated with SRS, the 5- and 10-year local tumor control rates were 98.5% and 97%, respectively.[39] Starke and colleagues[53] reported the outcomes of a cohort of 255 patients having skull base meningiomas treated with SRS. The 5- and 10-year reported local tumor control rates were 96% and 79%, respectively, with a 10% rate of neurologic deterioration.[53]

In a series of 199 meningiomas, located predominantly in the skull base treated with Cyberknife radiosurgery, the 5-year local tumor control was 93.5%. Tumors greater than 8 mL were treated with volume-staged multisession Cyberknife radiosurgery (2–5 sessions).[54] Cyberknife radiosurgery has also been reported for perioptic parasellar meningiomas by the Stanford group[55] with good results in terms of visual function preservation. Other technologies (Novalis TX or Gamma Knife Extend) are used to deliver multisession radiosurgery to perioptic parasellar meningiomas with comparable safety as well.

Convexity Meningiomas

Convexity meningiomas have historically been resected surgically or followed conservatively. A complete resection of the tumor, associated dura, and involved bone (Simpson's grade I), is curative in intent. With the success of SRS for skull base meningiomas, SRS indications have been extended and applied to convexity meningiomas in selected cases. Radiosurgical series treating convexity meningiomas typically demonstrate local tumor control rates comparable with that observed in skull base series. Still, SRS risks associated with the treatment of a convexity meningioma are different. These more frequently involve the development of a postradiosurgical cerebral edema or other adverse radiation effects as compared with cranial nerve injuries that can arise with skull base lesions.[35,55,56]

Kondziolka and colleagues[56] reported a series of 125 patients with convexity meningiomas treated with single session SRS. Reported tumor control rates were 92% for those treated with upfront radiosurgery and 97% for those treated with radiosurgery as an adjuvant treatment. The overall morbidity rate was 9.6% with 5% developing edema or adverse radiation effects.[56] The morbidity rate is comparable with the 10% complication rate noted in microsurgical series of convexity meningioma patients.[57] Girvigian and colleagues[58] reported a lesser rate of complications when the target volume was smaller and the margin dose was less than 14 Gy.[58]

Pamir and colleagues[59] reported a series of 43 patients with meningiomas involving the sagittal sinus, with a median follow-up of 46 months, and a median margin dose of 15 Gy. Tumor control was reported in 88%. Pamir and colleagues[59] recommended that radiosurgery be used as the upfront treatment for patients with small tumors invading the superior sagittal sinus and minimal mass effect. For those with larger tumors, tumor resection without violation of the sinus and major cortical draining veins followed by radiosurgery for any residual or recurrent tumor (adaptive hybrid surgery) is advocated.

RADIOSURGERY FOR ATYPICAL AND MALIGNANT MENINGIOMAS

Surgical resection continues to play a major role in the treatment of atypical or malignant meningiomas. By their very nature, histopathologic diagnosis and grading are important for the management of higher grade meningiomas (ie, meningiomas beyond grade I). Radiosurgery without or without external beam radiotherapy is increasingly being used after surgery in the treatment of aggressive meningiomas. Still, Hardesty and colleagues[60] recently reported a series of 228 atypical meningiomas and found no difference in recurrence rates between patients treated with adjuvant radiosurgery, adjuvant intensity modulated radiation therapy, and surgery alone.[60] Data regarding treatment outcomes for patients with aggressive meningiomas treated with radiosurgery is limited. Additionally, much of the existing data are based on series dating before 2000, when a major revision of the WHO criteria occurred.

Table 2 lists the major series of treatment for aggressive meningiomas with radiosurgery. Several reports allude to the fact that a WHO grade III diagnosis is the strongest predictor of recurrence and mortality in aggressive meningioma patients treated with surgery and gamma knife radiosurgery.[11,12] The WHO grade was found to be the only parameter significant on multivariate analysis for both recurrence and survival.[11,12] Other important parameters for survival and recurrence are tumor size, nuclear atypia, necrosis, and increased mitotic rate.[12] Patients most likely to benefit from adjuvant SRS are those with smaller tumors.

RADIOSENSITIVITY OF CRANIAL NERVES

Meningiomas, particularly those involving the skull base, are frequently adjacent to cranial nerves. Radiation injury to the cranial nerves is probably secondary to microangiopathy and small blood vessels obliteration and secondary damage to the protective Schwann cells layer. There is a significant difference in the potential radiation tolerance of various cranial nerves with pure sensory nerves (the optic and cochlear cranial nerves) showing the most radiosensitivity. This may be owing in part to the fact that both the optic and acoustic nerves are in effect central nervous system fiber tracts. These cranial nerves show limited capacity for recovery from any form of injury (mechanical from surgery, compressive from a tumor, or ionizing from radiation). These nerves are followed by the mixed function cranial nerves coursing through the parasellar region (the oculomotor, trochlear, trigeminal and abducens nerves, cranial nerves III–VI), and the lower posterior fossa located cranial nerves (the facial nerve and the lower cranial nerves IX–XII) tolerating a higher dose safely.

The radiosensitivity of the sensory cranial nerves may limit the dose given to meningiomas that are in close proximity to these. Although the precise dose tolerance of the cranial nerves is unclear, the anterior visual pathways seem to be able to tolerate a single maximal dose of radiation in the range of 10 to 12 Gy.[22,24,32,36,61,62] Patients harboring parasellar or tuberculum sellae meningiomas, evaluated for single fraction SRS, require a careful assessment of the distance between the optic nerve and the tumor. The risk of visual dysfunction is related to the volume and length of the optic apparatus receiving a dose higher than 8 Gy.[22,24,32,36,61,62] The optic apparatus seems to tolerate a dose of 8 to as high as 12 Gy to a 1% volume. However, this tolerance of the optic nerves to radiation may be lessened by prior radiation therapy or preexisting neural injury. Classical teaching mandated a minimum distance of 5 mm between a meningioma and the anterior optic apparatus (ie, optic nerve and chiasm) to achieve an optimal dose fall off. Current modern radiosurgical devices and treatment paradigms as well as the possibility for hypofractionated (multisession) SRS approaches have decreased this distance to nearly zero.

HYPOFRACTIONATED STEREOTACTIC RADIOSURGERY

Hypofractionated SRS serves to integrate the benefits of focused high-dose radiation and conformity typically associated with single-session SRS, with the benefits of repair and repopulation of adjacent normal tissues and the potential to enhance tumor cells damage by reoxygenation and redistribution to more sensitive phases of the cell cycle in between fractions.[63] In particular, hypofractionated SRS may help to overcome the limitations of single-session SRS associated with larger volume meningiomas and meningiomas that are in close proximity to critical structure for which a single session approach would convey too high of a dose to such structures.[55,64] Thus, the definition of SRS has been rewritten to encompass treatment delivery in 1 to 5 sessions.[65]

Hypofractionation to perioptic meningiomas allows for delivery of 19.5 in 3 fractions and 25 Gy in 5 fractions to the optic pathways while still conveying a low risk of optic neuropathy.[66] Similarly maximal doses of 23 Gy in 3 fractions and 31 Gy in 5 fractions are considered reasonable safe when delivered to the brainstem using hypofractionated SRS.[66] For many grade I meningiomas that may be positioned in the perioptic region, SRS in 3 to 5 fractions with a mean margin dose of 20 to 25 Gy conveys a favorable rate of tumor control and a low risk of radiation-induced cranial neuropathy. In our series of predominantly perioptic tumors delivering a mean margin dose of 19.7 Gy in 3 to 5 fractions, we observed no dysfunction in cranial nerve II and tumor regression in 33% of patients, with stability in the remainder.[63] In another series of 49 patients with perioptic lesions of whom 27 had meningiomas, tumor control was achieved in 94% of patients.[55] In that same series, 8 of 35 patients with preexisting visual deficits had improvement in their vision; only 1 patient experienced visual loss related to radiation-induced injury.[55] Spatial/volume-staged SRS serves as another tool in our armamentarium for treating larger lesions. Haselsberger and colleagues[67] reported 90% tumor control rates and no permanent neurologic deficiencies in a series of 20 patients with large skull base meningiomas of greater than 3 cm in diameter.[67] Thus, hypofractionated SRS may afford a favorable benefit-to-risk profile for the treatment of meningiomas close to radiation-sensitive critical structures or for larger volume meningiomas.

STEREOTACTIC RADIOSURGERY–INDUCED COMPLICATIONS

The radiosurgical procedure itself is not typically associated with any immediate or upfront risks or adverse responses. Patients may sometimes experience nausea and if a frame-based procedure is performed, transient headaches may occur. Stereotactic frame pin site infections are very rare. Radiosurgery-related complications have been reported in 3% to 40% of patients, with most report complications of in the range of 8%. These are usually segregated to approximately 5% permanent and 3% transient complications. Complications include neurologic deficits associated with adverse radiation effects (AREs) seen on follow-up neuro-imaging (eg, edema, necrosis, etc.). These may include symptoms such as headaches, focal neurologic signs or convulsions. Other complications include a partial or complete cranial nerve dysfunction.

Cranial nerve dysfunction is most commonly seen in those patients with parasellar or other skull base meningiomas. The most significant factor in cranial nerve deficit development is the length (volume) of the nerve irradiated, not the volume of tumor or the maximal dose. Tishler and colleagues[68] noted that the maximum dose delivered to cranial nerves was related to neurologic deficits in 29 patients after LINAC radiosurgery and 33 patients after gamma knife radiosurgery.[68] Doses up to 40 Gy were shown to be safe for the cranial nerves in the parasellar region. Our group previously reported a series of SRS for trigeminal neuralgia for a cohort of 151 patients, treated with 80 to 90 Gy to the cisternal segment of the trigeminal nerve. 12 patients (9%) developed new-onset facial numbness after SRS.[69] In treating patients with parasellar and sellar tumor histologies, we have delivered doses of 20 to 30 Gy to the cranial nerves in the parasellar region with only rare complications.[69]

Radiosurgical-induced changes (AREs) in the surrounding brain parenchyma after treatment of a meningioma have been well described, usually developing 8 to 18 months after the SRS treatment. Incidence reports vary, with one report noting an incidence of 24.7%.[70] Those with preexisting peritumoral edema or a larger tumor surface area were reported to be at a greater risk of developing worsening AREs.[70] Such changes may be associated with focal or diffuse neurologic sequelae and seizures, although many of these T2 weighted and postcontrast changes on MRI can be reversible. Increased risk of post-SRS AREs have been reported to be associated with various factors. These include age greater than 60 years, perilesional edema before radiosurgery,

no previous surgical resection, a larger treatment volume (eg, >10 mL), tumor location in the anterior cranial fossa, and a higher margin dose (eg, >15 Gy).[71]

SUMMERY: THE ROLE FOR STEREOTACTIC RADIOSURGERY IN THE MANAGEMENT OF MENINGIOMAS

In the past decades, SRS has been established as having a major role in the treatment for meningioma patients. SRS should be considered in certain tumor and patient related conditions. Although watchful follow-up can be advocated in certain cases, a growing lesion or one causing clinical symptoms merits consideration for a more aggressive approach. Still, when considering more aggressive treatment options, one should bear in mind the patient's life span, personal goals of care/expectations, and the widespread reduced tolerance to major postprocedural (postoperative) neurologic deficits, as compared with the past.

In a fit patient, meningiomas located in readily accessible regions, such as the convexity, parasagittal area, and sphenoid wing, may be more amenable to upfront surgical resection than SRS.[72] The incidence of SRS-induced AREs is higher with convexity, parasagittal and parafalcine meningiomas than with skull base meningiomas.[73,74] Large skull base meningiomas associated with symptomatic compression of critical neurovascular structures should be strongly considered for surgical debulking before radiation therapy.[75] The same holds true for lesions causing obstructive hydrocephalus. These should undergo initial surgical treatment for cerebrospinal fluid diversion.

SRS should be considered for benign meningiomas involving critical neuronal or vascular structures and for residual skull base tumors after microsurgery particularly in patients with a long life expectancy in which the residual meningioma is more likely to demonstrate growth. Meningioma growth is difficult to forecast, particularly on an individual patient basis. As such, follow-up of residual meningiomas not treated with radiosurgery should be performed in such a way that any growth of the residual tumor be detected before it exceed the typical volume constraints of radiosurgery thereby closing a valuable, less invasive (than resection) treatment window for the patient.

Alternatively, radiosurgery may be offered for patients not fit for major surgery (ie, those with significant comorbidities that make the person a high operative risk). In addition, radiosurgery can be used to treat meningiomas for those unwilling to accept the upfront risks of an open resection. Increasingly the attractiveness of less invasive options for treatment such as SRS in patients equally suited for resection or radiosurgery may make radiosurgery the treatment of choice for the patient's standpoint. The durability of response for SRS based on extensive literature makes this approach reasonable even for younger meningioma patients with a decade or more of life ahead.

In atypical or malignant meningiomas, SRS is generally viewed as a second tier treatment option, once surgical resection and/or conventional radiation have failed. In this challenging scenario for higher grade meningiomas, SRS seems to offer some clinical and tumor control benefit with a safe side effect profile.

REFERENCES

1. Deltour I, Johansen C, Auvinen A, et al. Time trends in brain tumor incidence rates in Denmark, Finland, Norway, and Sweden, 1974-2003. J Natl Cancer Inst 2009;101:1721–4.

2. Mawrin C, Perry A. Pathological classification and molecular genetics of meningiomas. J Neurooncol 2010;99:379–91.

3. Surawicz TS, McCarthy BJ, Kupelian V, et al. Descriptive epidemiology of primary brain and CNS tumors: results from the central brain tumor registry of the United States, 1990 – 1994. Neuro Oncol 1999;1:14–25.

4. Modha A, Gutin PH. Diagnosis and treatment of atypical and anaplastic meningiomas: a review. Neurosurgery 2005;57:538–50 [discussion: 538–50].

5. Bondy M, Ligon BL. Epidemiology and etiology of intracranial meningiomas: a review. J Neurooncol 1996;29:197–205.

6. Riemenschneider MJ, Perry A, Reifenberger G. Histological classification and molecular genetics of meningiomas. Lancet Neurol 2006;5:1045–54.

7. Louis DN, Ohgaki H, Wiestler OD, et al. The 2007 who classification of tumours of the central nervous system. Acta Neuropathol 2007;114:97–109.

8. Rogers L, Gilbert M, Vogelbaum MA. Intracranial meningiomas of atypical (WHO grade II) histology. J Neurooncol 2010;99:393–405.

9. Claus EB, Bondy ML, Schildkraut JM, et al. Epidemiology of intracranial meningioma. Neurosurgery 2005;57:1088–95 [discussion: 1088–95].

10. Pearson BE, Markert JM, Fisher WS, et al. Hitting a moving target: evolution of a treatment paradigm for atypical meningiomas amid changing diagnostic criteria. Neurosurg Focus 2008;24(5):E3.

11. Kaur G, Sayegh ET, Larson A, et al. Adjuvant radiotherapy for atypical and malignant meningiomas: a systematic review. Neuro Oncol 2014;16: 628–36.

12. Ferraro DJ, Funk RK, Blackett JW, et al. A retrospective analysis of survival and prognostic factors after stereotactic radiosurgery for aggressive meningiomas. Radiat Oncol 2014; 27(9):38.

13. Perry A, Scheithauer BW, Stafford SL, et al. "Malignancy" in meningiomas: a clinicopathologic study of 116 patients, with grading implications. Cancer 1999;85:2046–56.

14. Pasquier D, Bijmolt S, Veninga T, et al. Atypical and malignant meningioma: outcome and prognostic factors in 119 irradiated patients. A multicenter, retrospective study of the rare cancer network. Int J Radiat Oncol Biol Phys 2008;71: 1388–93.

15. Simpson D. The recurrence of intracranial meningiomas after surgical treatment. J Neurol Neurosurg Psychiatry 1957;20:22–39.

16. Arnautovic KI, Al-Mefty O, Husain M. Ventral foramen magnum meningiomas. J Neurosurg 2000;92: 71–80.

17. Couldwell WT, Fukushima T, Giannotta SL, et al. Petroclival meningiomas: surgical experience in 109 cases. J Neurosurg 1996;84:20–8.

18. Natarajan SK, Sekhar LN, Schessel D, et al. Petroclival meningiomas: multimodality treatment and outcomes at long-term follow-up. Neurosurgery 2007;60:965–81.

19. Mathiesen T, Gerlich A, Kihlstrom L, et al. Effects of using combined transpetrosal surgical approaches to treat petroclival meningiomas. Neurosurgery 2007;60:982–91 [discussion: 991–2].

20. Strang RD, Al-Mefty O. Comment on stereotactic radiosurgery for meningioma. In: Pollock BE, editor. Contemporary stereotactic radiosurgery: technique and evaluation. Armonk (NY): Futura Publishing; 2002. p. 172–80.

21. Sughrue ME, Kane AJ, Shangari G, et al. The relevance of Simpson grade I and II resection in modern neurosurgical treatment of World Health Organization grade I meningiomas. J Neurosurg 2010;113: 1029–35.

22. Seung SK, Larson DA, Galvin JM, et al. American college of radiology (ACR) and American Society for Radiation Oncology (ASTRO) practice guideline for the performance of stereotactic radiosurgery (SRS). Am J Clin Oncol 2006;36: 310–5.

23. Ding D, Yen CP, Starke RM, et al. Unyielding progress: recent advances in the treatment of central nervous system neoplasms with radiosurgery and radiation therapy. J Neurooncol 2014; 119:513–29.

24. Kirkpatrick JP, Meyer JJ, Marks LB. The linear-quadratic model is inappropriate to model high dose per fraction effects in radiosurgery. Semin Radiat Oncol 2008;18:240–3.

25. Garcia-Barros M, Paris F, Cordon-Cardo C, et al. Tumor response to radiotherapy regulated by endothelial cell apoptosis. Science 2003;300:1155–9.

26. Song CW, Cho LC, Yuan J, et al. Radiobiology of stereotactic body radiation therapy/stereotactic radiosurgery and the linear-quadratic model. Int J Radiat Oncol Biol Phys 2013;87(1):18–9.

27. Ma L, Larson D, Petti P, et al. Boosting central target dose by optimizing embedded dose hot spots for gamma knife radiosurgery. Stereotact Funct Neurosurg 2007;85:259–63.

28. Lee JY, Niranjan A, McInerney J, et al. Stereotactic radiosurgery providing long-term tumor control of cavernous sinus meningiomas. J Neurosurg 2002;97:65–72.

29. Iwai Y, Yamanaka K, Ikeda H. Gamma knife radiosurgery for skull base meningiomas: long-term results of low dose treatment. J Neurosurg 2008;109:804–10.

30. Pollock BE, Stafford SL, Utter A, et al. Stereotactic radiosurgery provides equivalent tumor control to Simpson grade 1 resection for patients with small-to medium-size meningiomas. Int J Radiat Oncol Biol Phys 2003;55:1000–5.

31. Ding D, Starke RM, Hantzmon J, et al. The role of radiosurgery in the management of WHO grade II and III intracranial meningiomas. Neurosurg Focus 2013;35:E16.

32. Sheehan JP, Williams BJ, Yen CP. Stereotactic radiosurgery for WHO grade I meningiomas. J Neurooncol 2010;99:407–16.

33. Ganz JC, Backlund EO, Thorsen FA. The results of gamma knife surgery of meningiomas, related to size of tumor and dose. Stereotact Funct Neurosurg 1993;61(Suppl 1):23–9.

34. Kondziolka D, Flickinger JC, Perez B. Judicious resection and/or radiosurgery for parasagittal meningiomas: outcomes from a multicenter review. Gamma knife meningioma study group. Neurosurgery 1998;43:405–13.

35. DiBiase SJ, Kwok Y, Yovino S, et al. Factors predicting local tumor control after gamma knife stereotactic radiosurgery for benign intracranial meningiomas. Int J Radiat Oncol Biol Phys 2004;60:1515–9.

36. Pollock BE, Stafford SL, Link MJ, et al. Single-fraction radiosurgery for presumed intracranial meningiomas: efficacy and complications from a 22-year experience. Int J Radiat Oncol Biol Phys 2012;83:1414–8.

37. Pollock BE, Stafford SL, Link MJ, et al. Stereotactic radiosurgery of World Health Organization grade II and III intracranial meningiomas: treatment results on the basis of a 22-year experience. Cancer 2012;118:1048–54.

38. Flickinger JC, Kondziolka D, Maitz AH, et al. Gamma knife radiosurgery of imaging-diagnosed intracranial meningioma. Int J Radiat Oncol Biol Phys 2003;56:801–6.

39. Kreil W, Luggin J, Fuchs I, et al. Long term experience of gamma knife radiosurgery for benign skull base meningiomas. J Neurol Neurosurg Psychiatry 2005;76:1425–30.

40. Starke RM, Nguyen JH, Rainey J, et al. Gamma knife surgery of meningiomas located in the posterior fossa: factors predictive of outcome and remission. J Neurosurg 2011;114:1399–409.

41. Kondziolka D, Levy EI, Niranjan A, et al. Long-term outcomes after meningioma radiosurgery: physician and patient perspectives. J Neurosurg 1999;91:44–50.

42. Henzel M, Gross MW, Hamm K, et al. Significant tumor volume reduction of meningiomas after stereotactic radiotherapy: results of a prospective multicenter study. Neurosurgery 2006;59:1188–94 [discussion: 1194].

43. Henzel M, Gross MW, Hamm K, et al. Stereotactic radiotherapy of meningiomas: symptomatology, acute and late toxicity. Strahlenther Onkol 2006;182:382–8.

44. Fokas E, Henzel M, Surber G, et al. Stereotactic radiation therapy for benign meningioma: long-term outcome in 318 patients. Int J Radiat Oncol Biol Phys 2014;89:569–75.

45. Starke RM, Przybylowski CJ, Sugoto M, et al. Gamma knife radiosurgery of large skull base meningiomas. J Neurosurg 2014;5:1–10.

46. Kondziolka D, Mathieu D, Lunsford LD, et al. Radiosurgery as definitive management of intracranial meningiomas. Neurosurgery 2008;62:53–60.

47. Santacroce A, Waller M, Regis J, et al. Long-term control of benign intracranial meningiomas after radiosurgery in a series of 4565 patients. Neurosurgery 2012;70:32–9.

48. Bledsoe JM, Link MJ, Stafford SL, et al. Radiosurgery for large-volume (> 10 cm3) benign meningiomas. J Neurosurg 2009;112:951–6.

49. Kondziolka D, Patel AD, Kano H, et al. Long-term outcomes after gamma knife radiosurgery for meningiomas. Am J Clin Oncol 2014 [Epub ahead of print].

50. Spiegelmann R, Cohen ZR, Nissim O, et al. Cavernous sinus meningiomas: a large LINAC radiosurgery series. J Neurooncol 2010;98:195–202.

51. Cohen-Inbar O, Lee CC, Schlesinger D, et al. Stereotactic radiosurgery for skull base meningiomas – long-term results. Neurosurgery 2015. [Epub ahead of print].

52. Starke R, Kano H, Ding D, et al. Stereotactic radiosurgery of petroclival meningiomas: a multicenter study. J Neurooncol 2014;119:169–76.

53. Starke RM, Williams BJ, Hiles C, et al. Gamma knife surgery for skull base meningiomas. J Neurosurg 2012;116:588–97.

54. Colombo F, Casentini L, Cavedon C, et al. Cyber-knife radiosurgery for benign meningiomas: short-term results in 199 patients. Neurosurgery 2009; 64(2 Suppl):A7–13.

55. Adler JR Jr, Gibbs IC, Puataweepong P, et al. Visual field preservation after multisession cyberknife radiosurgery for perioptic lesions. Neurosurgery 2006;59:244–54 [discussion: 244–54].

56. Kondziolka D, Madhok R, Lunsford LD, et al. Stereotactic radiosurgery for convexity meningiomas. J Neurosurg 2009;111:458–63.

57. Sanai N, Sughrue ME, Shangari G, et al. Risk profile associated with convexity meningioma resection in the modern neurosurgical era. J Neurosurg 2009; 112:913–9.

58. Girvigian MR, Chen JC, Rahimian J, et al. Comparison of early complications for patients with convexity and parasagittal meningiomas treated with either stereotactic radiosurgery or fractionated stereotactic radiotherapy. Neurosurgery 2008;62(5 Suppl):A19–27 [discussion: A27–8].

59. Pamir MN, Peker S, Kilic T, et al. Efficacy of gamma-knife surgery for treating meningiomas that involve the superior sagittal sinus. Zentralbl Neurochir 2007;68(2):73–8.

60. Hardesty DA, Wolf AB, Brachman DG, et al. The impact of adjuvant stereotactic radiosurgery on atypical meningioma recurrence following aggressive microsurgical resection. J Neurosurg 2013; 119:475–81.

61. Jagannathan J, Sheehan JP, Pouratian N, et al. Gamma knife surgery for Cushing's disease. J Neurosurg 2007;106(6):980–7.

62. Lawrence YR, Li XA, el Naqa I, et al. Radiation dose-volume effects in the brain. Int J Radiat Oncol Biol Phys 2010;76(3 Suppl):S20–7.

63. Nguyen JH, Chen CJ, Lee CC, et al. Multisession gamma knife radiosurgery: a preliminary experience with a non-invasive, relocatable frame. World Neurosurg 2014;82(6):1256–63.

64. Adler JR Jr, Gibbs IC, Puataweepong P, et al. Visual field preservation after multisession cyberknife radiosurgery for perioptic lesions. Neurosurgery 2008;62(Suppl 2):733–43.

65. Barnett GH, Linskey ME, Adler JR, et al. Stereotactic radiosurgery–an organized neurosurgery-sanctioned definition. J Neurosurg 2007;106(1):1–5.

66. Timmerman RD. An overview of hypofractionation and introduction to this issue of seminars in radiation oncology. Semin Radiat Oncol 2008;18(4): 215–22.

67. Haselsberger K, Maier T, Dominikus K, et al. Staged gamma knife radiosurgery for large critically located benign meningiomas: evaluation of a series comprising 20 patients. J Neurol Neurosurg Psychiatry 2009;80(10):1172–5.

68. Tishler RB, Loeffler JS, Lunsford LD, et al. Tolerance of cranial nerves of the cavernous sinus to radiosurgery. Int J Radiat Oncol Biol Phys 1993; 27:215–21.

69. Sheehan J, Pan HC, Stroila M, et al. Gamma knife surgery for trigeminal neuralgia: outcomes and prognostic factors. J Neurosurg 2005;102:434–41.

70. Cai R, Barnett GH, Novak E, et al. Principal risk of peritumoral edema after stereotactic radiosurgery for intracranial meningioma is tumor-brain contact interface area. Neurosurgery 2005;66: 513–22.

71. Kollova A, Liscak R, Novotny J Jr, et al. Gamma knife surgery for benign meningioma. J Neurosurg 2007; 107:325–36.

72. Sughrue ME, Rutkowski MJ, Chen CJ, et al. Modern surgical outcomes following surgery for sphenoid wing meningiomas. J Neurosurg 2013;119:86–93.

73. Chang JH, Chang JW, Choi JY, et al. Complications after gamma knife radiosurgery for benign meningiomas. J Neurol Neurosurg Psychiatry 2003;74:226–30.

74. Ding D, Xu Z, McNeill IT, et al. Radiosurgery for parasagittal and parafalcine meningiomas. J Neurosurg 2013;119:871–7.

75. Nanda A, Javalkar V, Banerjee AD. Petroclival meningiomas: study on outcomes, complications and recurrence rates. J Neurosurg 2011;114:1268–77.

76. Pollock BE, Stafford SL, Link MJ, et al. Single-fraction radiosurgery of benign intracranial meningiomas. Neurosurgery 2012;71:604–13.

77. Zada G, Pagnini P, Yu C, et al. Long-term outcomes and patterns of tumor progression after gamma knife radiosurgery of benign meningiomas. Neurosurgery 2010;67:322–9.

78. Stafford SL, Pollock BE, Foote RL, et al. Meningioma radiosurgery: tumor control, outcomes, and complications among 190 consecutive patients. Neurosurgery 2001;49:1029–37 [discussion: 1037–8].

79. Kim DG, Kim Ch H, Chung HT, et al. Gamma knife surgery of superficially located meningioma. J Neurosurg 2005;102(Suppl):255–8.

80. Williams BJ, Yen CP, Starke RM, et al. Gamma knife surgery for parasellar meningiomas: long-term results including complications, predictive factors, and progression-free survival. J Neurosurg 2011; 114:1571–7.

81. Skeie BS, Enger P, Skeie GO, et al. Gamma knife surgery of meningiomas involving the cavernous sinus: long-term follow-up of 100 patients. Neurosurgery 2010;66:661–9.

82. Hasegawa T, Kida Y, Yoshimoto M, et al. Long-term outcomes of gamma knife surgery for cavernous sinus meningioma. J Neurosurg 2007;107:745–51.

83. Nicolato A, Foroni R, Pellegrino M, et al. Gamma knife radiosurgery in meningiomas of the posterior fossa. Experience with 62 treated lesions. Minim Invasive Neurosurg 2001;44:211–7.

84. Starke RM, Nguyen J, Reames DL, et al. Gamma knife radiosurgery of meningiomas involving the foramen magnum. J Craniovertebr Junction Spine 2010;1:5.

85. Ojemann SG, Sneed PK, Larson DA, et al. Radiosurgery for malignant meningioma: results in 22 patients. J Neurosurg 2000;93(Suppl 3): 62–7.

86. Harris AE, Lee JYK, Omalu B, et al. The effect of radiosurgery during management of aggressive meningiomas. Surg Neurol 2003;60:298–305 [discussion: 305].

87. Huffmann BC, Reinacher PC, Gilsbach JM. Gamma knife surgery for atypical meningiomas. J Neurosurg 2005;102(Supp):283–6.

88. Attia A, Chan MD, Mott RT, et al. Patterns of failure after treatment of atypical meningioma with gamma knife radiosurgery. J Neurooncol 2012;108:179–85.

89. Mori Y, Tsugawa T, Hashizume C, et al. Gamma knife stereotactic radiosurgery for atypical and malignant meningiomas. Acta Neurochir Suppl 2013;116:85–9.

90. Tamura M, Kubo K, Okita R, et al. Management of non-benign meningiomas with gamma knife radiosurgery. Acta Neurochir Suppl 2013;116:91–7.

Incidental Meningiomas
Management in the Neuroimaging Era

Marko Spasic, MD[a], Panayiotis E. Pelargos, MS[a],
Natalie Barnette, BS[a], Nikhilesh S. Bhatt, BS[a],
Seung James Lee, BS[a], Nolan Ung, BS[a],
Quinton Gopen, MD[b], Isaac Yang, MD[a],*

KEYWORDS

- Meningiomas • Neuroimaging • MRI • Computed tomography

KEY POINTS

- The number of patient imaging studies has increased because of precautious physicians ordering scans when a vague symptom is presented; subsequently, the number of incidental meningiomas detected has increased as well.
- These brain tumors do not present with related symptoms and are usually small. MRI and computed tomographic scans most frequently capture incidental meningiomas.
- Incidental meningiomas are managed with observation, radiation, and surgical resection.
- Ultimately, a conservative approach is recommended, such as observing an incidental meningioma and then only radiating if the tumor displays growth, whereas a surgical approach is to be used only when proven necessary.
- A conservative approach for incidental meningiomas provides the highest quality of care for patients, because lives are not subject to costly, unnecessary procedures.

INTRODUCTION

Meningiomas arise from the arachnoid caps cells on the outer surface of the meninges and are the second most common primary brain tumor.[1–4] They account for 13% to 37% of all intracranial tumors.[2,5–7] These tumors are estimated to be seen in 97.5 per 100,000 individuals per year.[8,9] Diagnosis of meningiomas is more frequent in women. The Registry of the United States states that meningiomas are identified more than twice as frequently in female patients.[8,10] In addition, elderly patients are detected with meningiomas at a higher frequency.[11] The incidence rates for this tumor in 2002 for age groups of 20 to 34, 45 to 54, 65 to 74, and 85+ were 0.74, 4.89, 12.79, and 18.86 per 100,000 individuals per year, respectively.[8,10] The World Health Organization (WHO) has histologically classified meningiomas into 3 grades: grade I (begin), grade II (atypical), grade III (malignant or anaplastic).[12] The estimated prevalence of each grade is 75%, 20% to 35%, and 1% to 3%, respectively.[13–16]

Incidental meningiomas are meningiomas that are found unexpectedly and without related symptoms.[17,18] Physicians have seen an increase in diagnosed incidental meningiomas due to the expansive use of neuroimaging for "imaging checkups" and precautionary diagnostics.[2,5,8,11,18–31] In the past few years, more

a Department of Neurological Surgery, University of California Los Angeles, Box 956901, Los Angeles, CA 90095-6901, USA; b Department of Otolaryngology - Head and Neck Surgery, University of California Los Angeles, 10833 Le Conte Ave., CHS 62-132, Los Angeles, CA 90095, USA
* Corresponding author. Department of Neurosurgery, University of California Los Angeles, 300 Stein Plaza, Suite 562, 5th Floor Wasserman Building, Los Angeles, CA 90095-6901.
E-mail address: iyang@mednet.ucla.edu

Neurosurg Clin N Am 27 (2016) 229–238
http://dx.doi.org/10.1016/j.nec.2015.11.012
1042-3680/16/$ – see front matter © 2016 Elsevier Inc. All rights reserved.

asymptomatic meningiomas were found each year than symptomatic meningiomas.[2,32] **Table 1** lists the patient age and tumor characteristics for all English-language published articles between 2005 and 2015 that present asymptomatic meningioma data.

Treatment modalities for meningiomas include observation, radiotherapy, and surgery.[1,4,8,19,31,33] Observation consists of obtaining and comparing serial images in intervals ranging from every 3 months to annually. Radiotherapy attempts to cease the growth of intracranial lesions by providing focused radiation to the tumor.[12] Surgical intervention involves a craniotomy to obtain a gross total resection (GTR) or subtotal resection (STR) of the tumor.[34]

However, the optimal management strategy for incidental meningiomas is controversial.[3,8,19,24,29,32,35–39] Some physicians recommend a conservative approach, while others advocate for more aggressive methods.[38] The contingencies between styles are often valid. On one hand, reports demonstrate that 24% to 54% of meningiomas will show growth.[3,4,6,11,29,38–40] On the other hand, the natural history confirms that typical growth is very slow.[2,3,5,19,21,24,32,36,38,39] Should a conservative approach be adopted knowing that the growth of the tumor is very slow? Or should an aggressive strategy be implemented given that growth is likely? Thus, physicians are presented with conflicting opinions on how to manage incidental meningiomas.

This review aims to discuss what diagnostic images have captured incidental meningiomas as well as the management strategies for these newly found asymptomatic intracranial tumors.

DIAGNOSTIC NEUROIMAGING TECHNIQUES

On radiographic imaging, meningiomas present as a well-marginalized lobular sphered contour or, more rarely, as a flat-sheeted contour, termed en plaque.[41] Whether the tumor appears to be spherical or en plaque, both have a substantial dural base.[42] The meningioma often pushes against the brain matter but rarely invades the parenchyma.[43] The following details different neuroimaging studies and some specific reports of their uses.

MRI

MRI is the preferred neuroimaging technique for diagnosis and evaluation of meningiomas because soft tissues can be differentiated with high resolution, multiplanar views are possible, and 3-dimensional simulations are easily reconstructed.[43–47] The standard signal intensity of meningiomas is characterized by isointensity to hypointensity on the T1-weighted sequence and isointensity to hyperintensity on the T2-weighted sequence.[41] Injection of contrast, most often gadolinium, leads to homogenous uptake of the contrast agent by the meningioma, and thus, a bright enhancement is displayed.[48] Necrotic or calcified portions of the meningioma do not take up the contrast agent as readily; thus, a bright enhancement is not displayed. Calcified portions are best detected on computed tomography (CT), although MRI can identify calcified portions of the meningioma by isointensity to hypointensity on the T2-weighted sequence.[41] T2-weighted-fluid-attenuated inversion recovery (T2-FLAIR) aids in determining areas of edema associated with the meningioma by suppressing the signal of the surrounding CSF.[49] This enhancement is greatly valued when differentiating a markedly hyperintense lesion from surrounding edema.[49,50] Most meningiomas are not associated with edema because of their slow-growing nature, although atypical or malignant meningiomas grow at a faster rate, making edema more likely in these cases.[51] The T2-FLAIR is also essential in pinpointing the dural tail of the meningioma.[43] Given that one study found a dural tail in 72% of meningiomas, this outgrowth can cautiously be used as diagnostic evidence.[41,52] This characteristic feature can only be used cautiously because other tumors, such as glial tumors, metastases, and lymphoma, can also present with a dural tail.[41,52,53] In short, MRI studies with and without contrast are essential in assessing soft tissue physiology, associated edema, semi-characteristic dural tail, and relational location of meningiomas.

Computed Tomography

CT is another important neuroimaging study when analyzing meningiomas because this technique allows for improved imaging of the calcified structures. This imaging study is also more accessible and lower in cost than MRI. Intravenous administration of contrast, usually iridium or barium, leads to homogenous uptake of contrast agent, resulting in even further enhancement of meningiomas.[52] This increased enhancement improves diagnostic accuracy.[54] The disadvantages and advantages of MRI are complemented by the disadvantages and advantages of CT.[45] First, MRI poorly delineates calcified portions of intracranial lesions, whereas CT outlines calcifications.[54,55] Hardened regions are observed in roughly 20% to 30% of meningiomas. Second, en plaque meningiomas are often not seen on CT, whereas en plaque meningiomas emerge on MRI.[54] As such, CT and MRI complement each other during imaging of meningiomas.

Table 1
Patient age and tumor characteristics for asymptomatic meningiomas reported from from 2005 to 2015

Article	Number of Patients	Mean Age (y)	Tumor Size at Diagnosis	Location			
				Skull Ease, n (%)	Convexity, n (%)	Falx/Parasagittal, n (%)	Other, n (%)
Jadid et al,[2] 2015	65	66.6	Average size = 2.36 cm Largest dimension: 21 (32.3%) tumors <2 cm 44 (67.7%) tumors >2 cm	32 (49.2)	13 (20)	20 (30.8)	0 (0)
Zeng et al,[33] 2015	112	N/A	Median diameter = 3.75 cm (range: 1–6 cm) Largest dimension: 28 (25.0%) tumors <3 cm 38 (33.9%) tumors = 3–4 cm 27 (24.1%) tumors = 4–5 cm 10 (8.9%) tumors = 5–6 cm 9 (8.0%) tumors ≥6 cm	29 (25.9)	37 (33.0)	40 (35.8)	6 (5.4)
Salvetti et al,[3,4] 2013	42	53	Median volume = 4.0 mL (range: 0.23–17.0 mL) Largest dimension: 10 (23.8%) tumors <2 cm 7 (16.7%) tumors = 2–2.5 cm 8 (42.8%) tumors >2.5 cm 7 (16.7%) tumors unknown initial size	22 (52.4)	10 (23.8)	8 (19.0)	1 (2.4)
Jo et al,[19] 2011	154	59.2	Mean diameter = 1.70 cm (range: 0.7–4.0 cm)	31 (20.1)	51 (33.1)	52 (33.8)	20 (13.0)
Hashiba et al,[6] 2009	70	61.6	Mean volume = 10.4 cm³ (range: 0.63–69.2 cm³)	7 (10.0)	27 (38.6)	20 (28.6)	16 (22.9)
Nabika et al,[36] 2007	70	58.3	N/A	N/A	N/A	N/A	N/A
Vernooij et al,[18] 2007	18	63.3	N/A	N/A	N/A	N/A	N/A
Yano et al,[38] 2006	603	N/A	Mean diameter = 2.4 cm	N/A	N/A	N/A	N/A
Sonoda et al,[37] 2005	16	74.8[a]	Mean diameter = 2.5 cm (range: 1.4–5.0 cm)	6 (37.5)	3 (18.8)	4 (25.0)	3 (18.8)

[a] Article described only patients greater than 70 years old.

Single-Photon Emission Computed Tomography

Single-photon emission computed tomography (SPECT) supplements the information provided by MRI and CT. Predictions concerning the vital biological characteristics can be made using SPECT.[56–59] Thallium-201 (^{201}Tl) is absorbed with high intensity in all meningiomas, although different grades of meningioma retain ^{201}Tl at different rates.[56,57,60] More aggressive meningiomas, such as malignant or recurrent meningiomas, demonstrate a higher late-phase collection of [201]Tl.[58,60–63] Compared with ^{201}Tl, [99m]Technetium- ([99m]Tc-) labeled radiotracers have 140-keV γ-ray energy, high proton flux, higher spatial resolution, higher availability, and lower patient encumbrance, making it the optimal class of radiotracer.[56] ^{99m}Tc-methoxyisobutylisonitrile (MIBI) aids in estimating grade, vascularity, and viability of meningiomas.[56,64,65] Degree of malignancy and vascularity directly correlates with meningiomas' uptake of ^{99m}Tc-MIBI. As ^{99m}Tc-MIBI increases, the likelihood of malignancy and vascularity increase as well.[56,64] Viability is estimated by noting if a portion of the meningioma does not uptake the radiotracer, because inactive, apoptotic, or necrotic portions do not uptake ^{99m}Tc-MIBI.[56,65] In summary, SPECT offers additional biological characteristics of meningiomas that CT and MRI do not present.

MANAGEMENT
Surgical Resection

Surgical resection for meningioma is usually considered for patients who have tumor growth of greater than 1 cm^3 per year or patients who have a symptomatic meningioma.[8,21,39] Surgical resection may also be beneficial for asymptomatic meningiomas to prevent possible tumor growth that would make surgery more complicated.[8,29,33,66] Several studies also recommend young patients with easily accessible asymptomatic meningiomas to be considered for surgery.[2,35] Tumor location and behavior and the patient's age and quality of life must be thoroughly evaluated before deciding to undergo surgical resection because of the risk of complications, morbidity, and mortality in meningioma surgery.[8,21,31,67,68]

The Simpson grading system is commonly used to predict recurrence.[69,70] Although complete resection is ideal, Simpson grade I resection is not always achievable when avoiding possible risks associated with differing inherent traits of every tumor. Surgical resection can be performed more easily on tumors with cerebral hemispheric

location, smaller size, and no peritumoral edema.[33,68,71–73] Meningiomas located in the convex dura and cerebral falx underwent a higher Simpson I resection rate than tumors located in the parasagittal sinus.[33,66] Simpson I resection becomes increasingly difficult when the tumor is located closer to critical structures. Patients with convexity meningiomas had no postsurgical complications; however, in patients with meningiomas in the anterior cranial fossa, falx, tentorium, medial sphenoid ridge, parasellar region, and cerebellopontine regions, the rate of complications were significantly higher.[33,66]

Surgical resection of the relatively smaller sizes of asymptomatic meningiomas compared with the larger sizes of symptomatic meningiomas seems to have an impact on the low complication rate. Reinert and colleagues[66] reviewed 201 patients who underwent surgical resection of asymptomatic meningiomas (<3 cm) and reported a significantly lower complication rate for asymptomatic meningiomas (4.9%) compared with complication rate for symptomatic meningiomas (23.2%).[33]

The morbidity and mortality rates for the surgical resection are much more pronounced in elderly patients with meningioma.[38] Yano et al.[38] indicate a higher complication rate (9.3%) for patients older than 70 compared to younger patients (4.4%).[33] Similarly, Kuratsu and colleagues[24] report a significantly higher morbidity rate for patients older than 70 years (23.3%) than patients younger than 70 (3.5%). Nishizaki and colleagues[7] also observed a significant negative correlation between Glasgow Outcome Score (GOS) and patient age at the time of surgery. Awad and colleagues[20] also report 75 patients older than 60 years who were surgically treated for both symptomatic and asymptomatic meningioma with a mortality rate of 6.6% and a morbidity rate of 48%. This large amount of evidence suggests that decisions to undergo surgical resection for asymptomatic meningioma must be made carefully, especially for elderly patients. Other complications common to elderly patients, such as pneumonia, renal dysfunction, arrhythmia, deep venous thrombosis, and pulmonary embolus, are not directly associated with the tumor and the technique of the tumor resection but, rather, result secondarily to these patients' comorbidities.[8,31]

Patients with Simpson grade I and II resections had significantly higher median survival rates than patients with Simpson grade III and IV resections.[69,74] Zeng and colleagues[33] reviewed 88 patients with asymptomatic meningiomas whom have undergone surgical resection; 88.6% of these patients successfully received Simpson I resections, and 81 of these patients (92%) returned to normal work and life. A great GOS score was maintained in more patients younger than 60 (97%) than in patients older than 60 (75%). This study also indicates a lower postsurgical complication rate (13.6%) for asymptomatic meningiomas than symptomatic meningiomas (21.7%).

Early postoperative imaging (PI) is critical in patients showing adverse symptoms after surgery, whereas early PI is not as crucial for asymptomatic patients with easily accessible meningiomas.[75] A strong correlation between the extent of the resection and tumor recurrence is also suggested.[33] One study also concludes that routine imaging is not indicated for asymptomatic meningiomas that were completely removed.[76] Nakasu and colleagues[26] suggest that many patients with benign meningioma have already reached the inflection point, or the deceleration of tumor growth, but in one case demonstrated a benign tumor that grew 8 times in 79 months. Asymptomatic meningiomas should be monitored via imaging until the tumor can be safely assumed to have passed the inflection point.

Most incidental meningiomas should be examined through CT or MRI before deciding on surgical resection. The first re-examination should be within 3 months to rule out malignancy. The second re-examination should be at 6 months to look for tumor growth. If the examinations seem to rule out malignancy and growth, the patient should then continue be examined at 1-year intervals.[33,38]

Radiation

Although surgical resection is the treatment modality that is preferentially selected when meningiomas have been observed to display growth or be responsible for symptoms, in certain cases radiation will be opted for as a management strategy instead.[4,7,66,77] Stereotactic radiotherapy (SRT) and stereotactic radiosurgery (SRS) are 2 of the principal radiation treatments that are used.[78] Both SRT and SRS can be effectively used as primary or adjuvant treatments for brain tumors, because they are capable of precisely delivering radiation to a predetermined target and avoid damaging nearby healthy tissue.[78,79] It has been reported that the tumor control rates of meningiomas treated with SRS have ranged from 86% to 96%.[78,80–85] In regards to asymptomatic meningiomas, SRS and SRT are used when patients have lesions that are at an increased risk for growth, are located in anatomic locations with high surgical morbidity, have comorbidities that elevate risk for surgery, or are older than 65 years old.[8]

In asymptomatic meningiomas located in close proximity with vital neurologic structures, radiation is a viable treatment option that can be used pre-emptively to prevent the lesion from increasing in size.[4] By using radiation pre-emptively, the compression of sensitive anatomic structures can be avoided.[31] In addition, meningiomas located in anatomic locations where surgical resection is technically challenging and has high rates of complications are often suggested to be treated with radiation.[77] Two precise locations where there are increased complication and mortality rates for surgical resection and SRS are the cavernous sinus and petroclival junction.[77] The reported rate of complication for benign meningiomas located in the cavernous sinus is 24% and has been noted to have a mortality rate that ranges from 7% to 18%.[77,86,87] A study that analyzed the results of surgical resection for petroclival tumors found that of 110 patients only 57% underwent GTR and 90% of patients suffered permanent cranial nerve deficits.[77,88] Although surgical resection is the first treatment option because it can result in complete removal of a tumor, SRS has been displayed to produce comparable outcomes to surgery.[77] Five-year actuarial progression-free survival (PFS) found that the local control rates for SRS produced outcomes that were highly comparable to those achieved by surgical resection.[77]

Radiation is also a feasible therapeutic strategy when asymptomatic meningiomas are at a high risk for becoming symptomatic due to the presence of characteristics that indicate increased chances for growth.[6,27,31,39,89] A study by Sughrue and colleagues[31] extensively analyzed the natural history of asymptomatic meningiomas and discovered that a tumor with a growth rate of more than 10% a year and peritumoral T2 hyperintensity had a 92% chance of progressing to cause symptoms.[4] Another finding by Sughrue and colleagues[31] suggested that the location and initial size of the meningioma are also indicators of potential for symptom development due to an increase in size. For example, it was discovered that 61% of lesions located in the cavernous sinus increased after a median follow-up of 4.6 years.[4] Conversely, it was displayed that a lesion located in the sphenoid wing only caused symptoms in 5% of patients.[4,31] Furthermore, the location of an asymptomatic meningioma in the cerebellopontine angle and petroclival region has been noted to lead to the development of symptoms in 28% and 40% of patients, respectively.[4,31] Asymptomatic meningiomas with the aforementioned histologies or anatomic locations that indicate increased tendencies for growth and developing symptoms are, therefore, cases in which SRS can be an effective treatment option.

A recent retrospective study analyzed the efficacy of Gamma Knife surgery (GKS)—a form of radiation treatment—to prevent the progression of asymptomatic meningiomas.[4] The median age of the 42 patients with asymptomatic meningioma treated in the study was 53 years old and the median tumor volume for the study was 4.0 mL.[4] It was found that the 5-year PFS was 91.1%, and 54.8% of the tumors had a reduction in volume as a result of GKS treatment.[4] Thus, it was posited that GKS is likely responsible for decreasing the growth of asymptomatic meningioma and helps prevent the development of symptoms from the lesion.[4] Other studies that evaluated the use of GKS to treat benign meningioma discovered similar tumor control rates; namely, it has been reported that the tumor control rates for GKS range from 90% to 100% after 5 years and the 10-year tumor control rate is 95%.[79,90–92]

Because of a high prevalence of comorbidities and a natural decline in their physiologic capacity, elderly patients are at an elevated risk for adverse events following surgery.[93,94] A meta-analysis that examined the outcomes of surgery on elder populations found the combined incidence of complications was 20% and varied between 2.7% and 29.8%.[93,95] In another study that analyzed surgical resection for patients older than 70 years of age, it was found that the morbidity rate was 9.4%, which was higher than the morbidity rate of 4.4% reported for patients younger than 70.[19,38] Accordingly, noninvasive treatment modalities, such as SRS, can be viewed to have additional advantages when used to treat elderly patients.[93] A recent study by Kaul and colleagues[93] analyzed the use of linac-based fractionated SRT (FSRT) for the treatment of meningiomas in older patients (age ≥65 years). After reviewing 100 cases that fit the appropriate criteria, Kaul and colleagues[93] found that the 3-, 5-, and 10-year PFS rates for elderly patients treated with FSRT were 93.7%, 91.1%, and 82%, respectively. A similar study that analyzed a cohort of 121 patients age ≥70 years had comparable findings.[95] More precisely, after 3 years, it was found that for benign meningiomas in elderly patients treated with various forms of SRS, there was a local control rate of 98.3% and an overall survival of 92%.[96]

Observation

Several studies question if some incidental meningiomas should be treated with surgical resection or radiation therapy.[31,39] Treatment of any kind should be considered only when intervening clearly enhances the patient's quality of life. Physicians have adopted a conservative observation approach in light of this treatment mentality. Observation consists of obtaining serial imaging and regular follow-up appointments to confirm insignificant growth and no related symptoms.[31] If serial imaging shows significant growth or the patient presents with related symptoms, then intervention, such as surgical resection and/or radiation therapy, can be adopted.[31]

This conservative approach comes with benefits and drawbacks. Positively, costly and sometimes unnecessary surgeries and radiation can be prolonged or sometimes even sidestepped all together.[31] This refrainment from treatment also delays or sometimes even avoids the associated risks with surgery and radiation.[31] Negatively, a histologic diagnosis cannot be obtained if more aggressive management is not implemented. WHO grade II and III meningiomas may therefore continue to grow without appropriate therapy.[89] Furthermore, there is the possibility that symptoms can present between follow-up appointments.[6,27,31,39,89] Also, there is the subsequent chance that the meningioma could grow rapidly between serial images, eliminating radiation as a treatment option and leaving only surgery as the optimal course of treatment.[31,79,82]

A planned time frame of when serial images are obtained and follow-up appointments are made can assist in reducing these negative drawbacks. MRI with and without contrast should first be obtained 3 months after diagnosis, then 9 months after diagnosis, and then a year after diagnosis.[3,31] This technique by no means equates to a histologic diagnosis but can ultimately provide evidence for the estimated grade of the tumor. If the imaging shows substantial growth or the patient presents with clinical symptoms, then it suggests that this incidental meningioma is a more aggressive lesion and should warrant more aggressive treatment.[31] However, if the imaging does not show substantial growth or the patient does not present with clinical symptoms, then it provides evidence that this incidental meningioma is stable and repeat MRI with and without contrast should be continued every year or every other year thereafter.[3,31] This technique does not eliminate the possibility of rapid growth of the lesion, leading to compulsory surgical treatment. Although it does reduce the chance of this issue compared with less frequent imaging, this procedure can and should be amended based on patient specifics and physician experience.

Evidence for this plan is supported by several studies. After compiling a meta-analysis of the literature, Sughrue and colleagues[31] report that 51% of patients with untreated meningiomas 2.5 cm or smaller displayed no tumor growth on serial imaging, whereas an additional 26% showed only minimal growth (≤10%) on serial imaging, after an average of 4.6 years. Only 2% of patients with meningiomas 2 cm or smaller reported new or worsening symptoms during their clinical follow-ups. In addition, Olivero and colleagues[3] found that 78% of asymptomatic meningiomas with an average diameter of 2.19 cm did not display an increase in tumor size, whereas the other 22% of asymptomatic meningiomas with an average diameter of 1.17 cm did display growth. The average growth rate was 0.24 cm per year. The ages between these groups only differed by 2.8 years. None of these patients developed symptoms over the course of the average 32 months of clinical follow up.

In summary, an overwhelming majority of the time small meningiomas hardly increase in size. In the instance that some growth does occur, only a small fraction of patients develop outward indications. These findings do not vary greatly between age groups. Given these statements, it is logical to follow an incidentally-detected small meningioma with serial imaging before proceeding with surgery or radiation.

SUMMARY

The number of patient imaging studies has increased because of precautious physicians ordering scans when a vague symptom is presented. Subsequently, the number of incidental meningiomas detected has increased as well. These brain tumors do not present with related symptoms and are usually small. MRI and CT scans most frequently capture incidental meningiomas. SPECT studies could then be used to gain further insight about important biological characteristics. After detection, a designated management strategy must be determined.

Incidental meningiomas can be managed with either observation, radiation, or surgical resection or any combination of these three. Each strategy is more advantageous for a particular circumstance. Observation requires serial imaging and clinical follow-ups and is best for small tumors that have shown no growth on repeated scans. SRS and SRT use focused beams of radiation to stunt tumor growth during a single sitting (SRS) or multiple fractions (SRT) and are best for small tumors that have shown minimal growth. Surgical resection aims for GTR or STR of the meningioma; this is best for large tumors or tumors in which the slightest growth could be detrimental.

Ultimately, a conservative approach is recommended, such as observing an incidental meningioma and then only radiating if the tumor displays growth, whereas a surgical approach is to be used only when proven necessary. A conservative approach for incidental meningiomas provides the highest quality of care for patients, because they are not subjected to costly, unnecessary procedures.

REFERENCES

1. Collins IM, Beddy P, O'Byrne KJ. Radiological response in an incidental meningioma in a patient treated with chemotherapy combined with CP-751,871, an IGF-1R inhibitor. Acta Oncol 2010; 49(6):872–4.
2. Jadid KD, Feychting M, Hoijer J, et al. Long-term follow-up of incidentally discovered meningiomas. Acta Neurochir 2015;157(2):225–30.
3. Olivero WC, Lister JR, Elwood PW. The natural history and growth rate of asymptomatic meningiomas: a review of 60 patients. J Neurosurg 1995; 83(2):222–4.
4. Salvetti DJ, Nagaraja TG, Levy C, et al. Gamma Knife surgery for the treatment of patients with asymptomatic meningiomas. J Neurosurg 2013; 119(2):487–93.
5. Chamberlain MC, Barnholtz-Sloan JS. Medical treatment of recurrent meningiomas. Expert Rev Neurother 2011;11(10):1425–32.
6. Hashiba T, Hashimoto N, Izumoto S, et al. Serial volumetric assessment of the natural history and growth pattern of incidentally discovered meningiomas. J Neurosurg 2009;110(4):675–84.
7. Nishizaki T, Ozaki S, Kwak T, et al. Clinical features and surgical outcome in patients with asymptomatic meningiomas. Br J Neurosurg 1999;13(1):52–5.
8. Chamoun R, Krisht KM, Couldwell WT. Incidental meningiomas. Neurosurg Focus 2011;31(6):E19.
9. Davis FG, Kupelian V, Freels S, et al. Prevalence estimates for primary brain tumors in the United States by behavior and major histology groups. Neuro Oncol 2001;3(3):152–8.
10. Claus EB, Bondy ML, Schildkraut JM, et al. Epidemiology of intracranial meningioma. Neurosurgery 2005;57(6):1088–95 [discussion: 1088–95].
11. Niiro M, Yatsushiro K, Nakamura K, et al. Natural history of elderly patients with asymptomatic meningiomas. J Neurol Neurosurg Psychiatry 2000;68(1): 25–8.
12. Kaur G, Sayegh ET, Larson A, et al. Adjuvant radiotherapy for atypical and malignant meningiomas: a systematic review. Neuro Oncol 2014;16(5):628–36.
13. Rogers L, Gilbert M, Vogelbaum MA. Intracranial meningiomas of atypical (WHO grade II) histology. J Neurooncol 2010;99(3):393–405.

14. Durand A, Labrousse F, Jouvet A, et al. WHO grade II and III meningiomas: a study of prognostic factors. J neuro-oncology 2009;95(3):367–75.

15. Zhou P, Ma W, Yin S, et al. Three risk factors for WHO grade II and III meningiomas: a study of 1737 cases from a single center. Neurol India 2013;61(1):40–4.

16. Aghi MK, Carter BS, Cosgrove GR, et al. Long-term recurrence rates of atypical meningiomas after gross total resection with or without postoperative adjuvant radiation. Neurosurgery 2009;64(1):56–60 [discussion: 60].

17. Illes J, Kirschen MP, Edwards E, et al. Ethics. Incidental findings in brain imaging research. Science 2006;311(5762):783–4.

18. Vernooij MW, Ikram MA, Tanghe HL, et al. Incidental findings on brain MRI in the general population. N Engl J Med 2007;357(18):1821–8.

19. Jo KW, Kim CH, Kong DS, et al. Treatment modalities and outcomes for asymptomatic meningiomas. Acta Neurochir (Wien) 2011;153(1):62–7 [discussion: 67].

20. Awad IA, Kalfas I, Hahn JF, et al. Intracranial meningiomas in the aged: surgical outcome in the era of computed tomography. Neurosurgery 1989;24(4): 557–60.

21. Couldwell WT. Asymptomatic meningiomas. J Neurosurg 2006;105(4):536–7 [discussion: 537].

22. Go RS, Taylor BV, Kimmel DW. The natural history of asymptomatic meningiomas in Olmsted County, Minnesota. Neurology 1998;51(6):1718–20.

23. Hashimoto N, Rabo CS, Okita Y, et al. Slower growth of skull base meningiomas compared with non-skull base meningiomas based on volumetric and biological studies. J Neurosurg 2012;116(3):574–80.

24. Kuratsu J, Kochi M, Ushio Y. Incidence and clinical features of asymptomatic meningiomas. J Neurosurg 2000;92(5):766–70.

25. Mantle RE, Lach B, Delgado MR, et al. Predicting the probability of meningioma recurrence based on the quantity of peritumoral brain edema on computerized tomography scanning. J Neurosurg 1999;91(3):375–83.

26. Nakasu S, Fukami T, Nakajima M, et al. Growth pattern changes of meningiomas: long-term analysis. Neurosurgery 2005;56(5):946–55 [discussion: 946–5].

27. Nakasu S, Nakasu Y, Fukami T, et al. Growth curve analysis of asymptomatic and symptomatic meningiomas. J Neurooncol 2011;102:310.

28. Onizuka M, Suyama K, Shibayama A, et al. Asymptomatic brain tumor detected at brain check-up. Neurol Med Chir (Tokyo) 2001;41(9):431–4 [discussion: 435].

29. Oya S, Kim S-H, Sade B, et al. The natural history of intracranial meningiomas. J Neurosurg 2011;114(5): 1250–6.

30. Radhakrishnan K, Mokri B, Parisi JE, et al. The trends in incidence of primary brain tumors in the population of Rochester, Minnesota. Ann Neurol 1995;37(1):67–73.

31. Sughrue ME, Rutkowski MJ, Aranda D, et al. Treatment decision making based on the published natural history and growth rate of small meningiomas. J Neurosurg 2010;113(5):1036–42.

32. Nakamura M, Roser F, Michel J, et al. The natural history of incidental meningiomas. Neurosurgery 2003;53(1):62–70 [discussion: 70–1].

33. Zeng L, Wang L, Ye F, et al. Clinical characteristics of patients with asymptomatic intracranial meningiomas and results of their surgical management. Neurosurg Rev 2015;38(3):481–8.

34. Veeravagu A, Azad TD, Chang SD. Perspective on "the role of adjuvant radiotherapy after gross total resection of atypical meningiomas". World Neurosurg 2015;83(5):737–8.

35. Herscovici Z, Rappaport Z, Sulkes J, et al. Natural history of conservatively treated meningiomas. Neurology 2004;63(6):1133–4.

36. Nabika S, Kiya K, Satoh H, et al. Strategy for the treatment of incidental meningiomas. No Shinkei Geka 2007;35(1):27–32 [in Japanese].

37. Sonoda Y, Sakurada K, Saino M, et al. Multimodal strategy for managing meningiomas in the elderly. Acta Neurochir (Wien) 2005;147(2):131–6 [discussion: 136].

38. Yano S, Kuratsu J, Kumamoto Brain Tumor Research Group. Indications for surgery in patients with asymptomatic meningiomas based on an extensive experience. J Neurosurg 2006;105(4):538–43.

39. Yoneoka Y, Fujii Y, Tanaka R. Growth of incidental meningiomas. Acta Neurochir (Wien) 2000;142(5): 507–11.

40. Iwai Y, Yamanaka K, Morikawa T, et al. The treatment for asymptomatic meningiomas in the era of radiosurgery. No Shinkei Geka 2003;31(8):891–7 [in Japanese].

41. Watts J, Box G, Galvin A, et al. Magnetic resonance imaging of meningiomas: a pictorial review. Insights Imaging 2014;5(1):113–22.

42. Buetow MP, Buetow PC, Smirniotopoulos JG. Typical, atypical, and misleading features in meningioma. Radiographics 1991;11(6):1087–106.

43. Islam OH, Grayson, Coombs B, et al. Imaging in brain meningioma. 2014. Available at: http://emedicine. medscape.com/article/341624-overview. Accessed September 8, 2015.

44. Morrison MC, Weiss KL, Moskos MM. CT and MR appearance of a primary intraosseous meningioma. J Comput Assist Tomogr 1988;12(1):169–70.

45. Schubeus P, Schorner W, Rottacker C, et al. Intracranial meningiomas: how frequent are indicative findings in CT and MRI? Neuroradiology 1990; 32(6):467–73.

46. Yamada S, Taoka T, Nakagawa I, et al. A magnetic resonance imaging technique to evaluate tumor-brain

adhesion in meningioma: brain-surface motion imaging. World Neurosurg 2015;83(1):102–7.

47. Yuan YQ, Hou M, Wu H, et al. A meningioma with peripheral rim enhancement on MRI. Brain Tumor Pathol 2012;29(4):235–9.

48. Chowdhury RW, Iain W, Rofe C, et al. Radiology at a glance. Hoboken, NJ: Wiley-Blackwell; 2010.

49. Husstedt HW, Sickert M, Kostler H, et al. Diagnostic value of the fast-FLAIR sequence in MR imaging of intracranial tumors. Eur Radiol 2000;10(5):745–52.

50. Hajnal JV, De Coene B, Lewis PD, et al. High signal regions in normal white matter shown by heavily T2-weighted CSF nulled IR sequences. J Comput Assist Tomogr 1992;16(4):506–13.

51. Eastmen GW, Wald C, Crossin J. Getting started in clinical radiology: from image to diagnosis. Stuttgart, Germany: Thieme; 2006.

52. O'Leary S, Adams WM, Parrish RW, et al. Atypical imaging appearances of intracranial meningiomas. Clin Radiol 2007;62(1):10–7.

53. Hakyemez B, Yildirim N, Erdogan C, et al. Meningiomas with conventional MRI findings resembling intraaxial tumors: can perfusion-weighted MRI be helpful in differentiation? Neuroradiology 2006; 48(10):695–702.

54. Kholsa AC, Bernard, DeLaPaz R, et al. Brain metastasis imaging. 2013. Available at: http://emedicine.medscape.com/article/338239-overview. Accessed August 2, 2015.

55. de la Sayette V, Rivaton F, Chapon F, et al. Meningioma of the third ventricle. Computed tomography and magnetic resonance imaging. Neuroradiology 1991;33(4):354–6.

56. Valotassiou V, Leondi A, Angelidis G, et al. SPECT and PET imaging of meningiomas. ScientificWorldJournal 2012;2012:412580.

57. Jinnouchi S, Hoshi H, Ohnishi T, et al. Thallium-201 SPECT for predicting histological types of meningiomas. J Nucl Med 1993;34(12):2091–4.

58. Tedeschi E, Soricelli A, Brunetti A, et al. Different thallium-201 single-photon emission tomographic patterns in benign and aggressive meningiomas. Eur J Nucl Med 1996;23(11):1478–84.

59. Kinuya K, Ohashi M, Itoh S, et al. Thallium-201 brain SPECT to diagnose aggressiveness of meningiomas. Ann Nucl Med 2003;17(6):463–7.

60. Matano F, Adachi K, Murai Y, et al. Microcystic meningioma with late-phase accumulation on thallium-201 single-photon emission computed tomography: case report. Neurol Med Chir 2014;54(8):686–9.

61. Black KL, Hawkins RA, Kim KT, et al. Use of thallium-201 SPECT to quantitate malignancy grade of gliomas. J Neurosurg 1989;71(3):342–6.

62. Ishibashi M, Taguchi A, Sugita Y, et al. Thallium-201 in brain tumors: relationship between tumor cell activity in astrocytic tumor and proliferating cell nuclear antigen. J Nucl Med 1995;36(12):2201–6.

63. Takeda T, Nakano T, Asano K, et al. Usefulness of thallium-201 SPECT in the evaluation of tumor natures in intracranial meningiomas. Neuroradiology 2011;53(11):867–73.

64. Bagni B, Pinna L, Tamarozzi R, et al. SPET imaging of intracranial tumours with 99Tcm-sestamibi. Nucl Med Commun 1995;16(4):258–64.

65. Ak I, Gulbas Z, Altinel F, et al. Tc-99m MIBI uptake and its relation to the proliferative potential of brain tumors. Clin Nucl Med 2003;28(1):29–33.

66. Reinert M, Babey M, Curschmann J, et al. Morbidity in 201 patients with small sized meningioma treated by microsurgery. Acta Neurochir (Wien) 2006; 148(12):1257–65 [discussion: 1266].

67. Bassiouni H, Hunold A, Asgari S, et al. Tentorial meningiomas: clinical results in 81 patients treated microsurgically. Neurosurgery 2004;55(1):108–16 [discussion: 116–8].

68. Sanai N, Sughrue ME, Shangari G, et al. Risk profile associated with convexity meningioma resection in the modern neurosurgical era. J Neurosurg 2010; 112(5):913–9.

69. Hammouche S, Clark S, Wong AH, et al. Long-term survival analysis of atypical meningiomas: survival rates, prognostic factors, operative and radiotherapy treatment. Acta Neurochir (Wien) 2014; 156(8):1475–81.

70. Simpson D. The recurrence of intracranial meningiomas after surgical treatment. J Neurol Neurosurg Psychiatry 1957;20(1):22–39.

71. Markovic M, Antunovic V, Milenkovic S, et al. Prognostic value of peritumoral edema and angiogenesis in intracranial meningioma surgery. J BUON 2013; 18(2):430–6.

72. Miao Y, Lu X, Qiu Y, et al. A multivariate analysis of prognostic factors for health-related quality of life in patients with surgically managed meningioma. J Clin Neurosci 2010;17(4):446–9.

73. Morokoff AP, Zauberman J, Black PM. Surgery for convexity meningiomas. Neurosurgery 2008;63(3): 427–33 [discussion: 433–4].

74. Zaher A, Abdelbari Mattar M, Zayed DH, et al. Atypical meningioma: a study of prognostic factors. World Neurosurg 2013;80(5):549–53.

75. Gebler FD, Dützmann S, Quick J, et al. Is postoperative imaging mandatory after meningioma removal? Results of prospective study. PLoS One 2015;10(4): e0124534.

76. Hodgson TJ, Kingsley DP, Moseley IF. The role of imaging in the follow up of meningiomas. J Neurol Neurosurg Psychiatry 1995;59(5):545–7.

77. Bloch O, Kaur G, Jian BJ, et al. Stereotactic radiosurgery for benign meningiomas. J neuro-oncology 2012;107(1):13–20.

78. Mansouri A, Larjani S, Klironomos G, et al. Predictors of response to Gamma Knife radiosurgery for intracranial meningiomas. J Neurosurg 2015;3:1–7.

79. Kondziolka D, Levy EI, Niranjan A, et al. Long-term outcomes after meningioma radiosurgery: physician and patient perspectives. J Neurosurg 1999;91(1): 44–50.

80. Igaki H, Maruyama K, Koga T, et al. Stereotactic radiosurgery for skull base meningioma. Neurol Med Chir 2009;49(10):456–61.

81. Kondziolka D, Flickinger JC, Perez B. Judicious resection and/or radiosurgery for parasagittal meningiomas: outcomes from a multicenter review. Gamma Knife Meningioma Study Group. Neurosurgery 1998;43(3):405–13 [discussion: 413–4].

82. Kondziolka D, Mathieu D, Lunsford LD, et al. Radiosurgery as definitive management of intracranial meningiomas. Neurosurgery 2008;62(1):53–8 [discussion: 58–60].

83. Korah MP, Nowlan AW, Johnstone PA, et al. Radiation therapy alone for imaging-defined meningiomas. Int J Radiat Oncol Biol Phys 2010;76(1): 181–6.

84. Pollock BE. Stereotactic radiosurgery for intracranial meningiomas: indications and results. Neurosurg Focus 2003;14(5):e4.

85. Pollock BE, Stafford SL. Results of stereotactic radiosurgery for patients with imaging defined cavernous sinus meningiomas. Int J Radiat Oncol Biol Phys 2005;62(5):1427–31.

86. DEMonte FS, Smith HK, Al-Mefty O. Outcome of aggressive removal of cavernous sinus meningiomas. J Neurosurg 1994;81(2):245–51.

87. O'Sullivan MG, van Loveren HR, Tew JM Jr. The surgical resectability of meningiomas of the cavernous sinus. Neurosurgery 1997;40(2):238–44 [discussion: 245–7].

88. Roberti F, Sekhar LN, Kalavakonda C, et al. Posterior fossa meningiomas: surgical experience in 161 cases. Surg Neurol 2001;56(1):8–20 [discussion: 20–1].

89. Pollock BE, Stafford SL, Utter A, et al. Stereotactic radiosurgery provides equivalent tumor control to Simpson Grade 1 resection for patients with small- to medium-size meningiomas. Int J Radiat Oncol Biol Phys 2003;55(4):1000–5.

90. Kondziolka D, Patel AD, Kano H, et al. Long-term outcomes after gamma knife radiosurgery for meningiomas. Am J Clin Oncol 2014. [Epub ahead of print].

91. Flickinger JC, Kondziolka D, Maitz AH, et al. Gamma knife radiosurgery of imaging-diagnosed intracranial meningioma. Int J Radiat Oncol Biol Phys 2003; 56(3):801–6.

92. Lee JY, Niranjan A, McInerney J, et al. Stereotactic radiosurgery providing long-term tumor control of cavernous sinus meningiomas. J Neurosurg 2002; 97(1):65–72.

93. Kaul D, Budach V, Graaf L, et al. Outcome of elderly patients with meningioma after image-guided stereotactic radiotherapy: a study of 100 cases. Biomed Res Int 2015;2015:868401.

94. Poon MT, Fung LH, Pu JK, et al. Outcome of elderly patients undergoing intracranial meningioma resection–a systematic review and meta-analysis. Br J Neurosurg 2014;28(3):303–9.

95. Fokas E, Henzel M, Surber G, et al. Stereotactic radiotherapy of benign meningioma in the elderly: clinical outcome and toxicity in 121 patients. Radiother Oncol 2014;111(3):457–62.

96. Bertagna F, Bosio G, Pinelli L, et al. Incidental 11C-choline PET/CT brain uptake due to meningioma in a patient studied for prostate cancer: correlation with MRI and imaging fusion. Clin Nucl Med 2013;38(11):e435–437.

Management of Atypical and Anaplastic Meningiomas

Simon Buttrick, MD, Ashish H. Shah, MD,
Ricardo J. Komotar, MD, Michael E. Ivan, MD, MBS*

KEYWORDS

- Malignant meningioma • Atypical meningioma • Anaplastic meningioma • Malignant meningioma
- Radiation therapy • Chemotherapy • Recurrence

KEY POINTS

- Since adoption of the 2007 World Health Organization (WHO) grading scheme, the number of meningiomas classified as WHO II or III has risen sharply.
- Despite aggressive treatment of malignant meningiomas, the average reported 5-year survival rates are in the range of 30% to 60%.
- Obtaining a gross total resection via surgery remains the best first-line treatment toward overall survival; however, in most patients, adjuvant radiotherapy is also recommended.
- Predictors of overall survival include tumor size, age, location, and histopathologic findings.
- New insights into the biological basis of meningioma growth have identified several exciting targeted therapeutic interventions that have shown promise toward improving the current pharmacologic treatment options.

INTRODUCTION

Although meningiomas are generally thought of as benign lesions, a substantial proportion displays more aggressive behavior.[1] These tumors are classified as atypical (World Health Organization [WHO] grade II) or anaplastic (WHO grade III) meningiomas. Their quoted incidence varies widely from 1.5% to 35% of all meningiomas, largely related to inconsistencies in histopathologic grading.[2,3] When the new WHO grading system is applied, the number likely lies closer to the higher end of this range. Among these high-grade meningiomas, atypical meningiomas outnumber anaplastic meningiomas by about 6

to 1.[3] High-grade meningiomas can arise either de novo or progress from lower grade tumors.[1] Whereas completely resected benign meningiomas have a relatively low risk of recurrence of approximately 10%, atypical and anaplastic meningiomas are characteristically more aggressive in nature and are associated with higher recurrence risks of 29% to 52 % and 50% to 94 %, respectively.[5,6] Unlike benign meningiomas, which seem to be linked to estrogen levels and are more common in women, atypical and anaplastic meningiomas are more common among men. They also seem to have a greater predilection for the cerebral convexities.

Disclosures: None.
Department of Neurosurgery, University of Miami, 2nd Floor, 1095 Northwest 14 Terrace D4-6, Miami, FL 33136, USA
* Corresponding author.
E-mail address: MIvan@med.miami.edu

Neurosurg Clin N Am 27 (2016) 239–247
http://dx.doi.org/10.1016/j.nec.2015.11.003

Surgery remains a mainstay of treatment of meningiomas that have either grown since previous imaging or those that produce symptoms. Typically, neurosurgeons aim for Simpson grade 1 resection (gross total resection [GTR] with excision of the dural tail and overlying invaded cranium). If a GTR is not attainable, clinicians may opt for a subtotal resection (STR) and adjuvant radiotherapy. The decision to use adjuvant radiation therapy (RT) is based on the extent of resection and the histologic tumor characteristics, and is generally added in cases of atypical and anaplastic meningiomas.[5,7] Unfortunately, when patients fail to respond to this standard initial therapy, current treatment options are extremely limited and the morbidity and mortality among these patients increases significantly due to neurologic deterioration secondary to aggressive growth, compression of neural structured by the tumor, and peritumoral edema.

Aided by rapid advances in biotechnology, understanding of meningiomas at the molecular level has grown vastly in recent years. With this, interest in targeted therapies has emerged in an effort to treat aggressive meningiomas that have failed traditional therapy. Results of many of these studies have been sobering but drugs such as everolimus and bevacizumab have shown some promise. Several clinical trials are ongoing and will, it is hoped, soon add to the armamentarium against this resilient disease.

PATIENT EVALUATION OVERVIEW

The clinical presentation of atypical and anaplastic meningiomas is similar to their benign counterparts and there are few clues to their more aggressive nature before tissue is obtained. Common symptoms include headaches, seizures, and focal neurologic deficits related to the location of the tumor. Paralleling the increasing use of diagnostic imaging, many tumors are also diagnosed incidentally.

As previously mentioned, estrogen does not seem to play as much of a role in the pathogenesis of high-grade meningiomas as it does in benign meningiomas. In fact, opposite to benign meningiomas, which have a higher incidence in female patients, the incidence of atypical and anaplastic meningiomas is doubled in male patients.[8] The one environmental factor consistently associated with atypical and anaplastic meningiomas is ionizing radiation, especially in younger patients. There are several reports of patients who received cranial irradiation for various tumors and later went on to develop high-grade radiation-induced meningiomas.[9]

To date, there are no reliable radiologic indicators of malignancy in meningiomas. Several features on MRI, including increased peritumoral edema, heterogeneous appearance, hyperintensity on diffusion-weighted imaging, and characteristic fluid-attenuated inversion-recovery (FLAIR) appearance of the brain-meningioma interface, have been found to have some predictive value. However, all these features can also be seen in benign meningioma[9,10] (**Fig. 1**). Magnetic resonance spectroscopy has been used in small studies, showing increased lipid and lactate peaks in nonbenign meningiomas, but more work is needed to validate this and to assess what the role of this method might be in clinical practice.[11]

Location of the tumor has been shown to correlate with a patient's chance of both recurrence and atypia. One group of investigators has identified that a non–skull base location increased the risk for grade II or III disease by twofold.[8] Additionally, skull base location was associated with longer progression-free survival in atypical meningiomas.

Though Cushing[12,13] recognized the malignant potential of meningiomas in the 1930s, no uniform grading system gained widespread acceptance until the year 2000. In the 1990s, the Mayo clinic group proposed a set of criteria for atypical and anaplastic meningiomas based on analysis of their large series, which demonstrated that, in the absence of frank anaplasia, brain invasion was a highly significant predictor of recurrence risk, even in otherwise histologically benign appearing tumors.[14] This prompted the inclusion of brain invasion as one of the criteria for atypical meningiomas and significantly increased the number of tumors now classified as such. Based on these findings, WHO adopted the current 2007 uniform grading criteria for atypical and anaplastic meningiomas, summarized in **Table 1**.[15] Given the changes in the WHO classification, the authors have attempted to generate data from resources published in the last 10 years. This encompasses data during the changes of the WHO classification from 2000 to 2007.

Histochemical profiles of atypical and anaplastic meningioma are similar to WHO grade I meningiomas. These markers include epithelial membrane antigen (EMA) and vimentin positivity, and negative or weak staining for S-100 protein. Histologically, anaplasia seems to be the most significant risk factor for early mortality. In the aforementioned Mayo clinic series, median survival for frankly anaplastic meningiomas was only 1.5 years. Among tumors with brain invasion but without anaplasia, median survival was 14.9 years with otherwise benign morphology and 10.4 years with atypical morphology. This difference did not

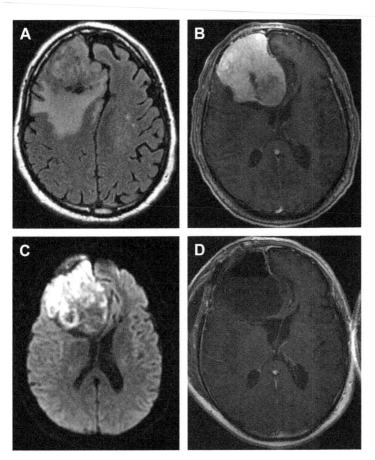

Fig. 1. Axial MRI findings of a patient with an atypical meningioma of the right frontal lobe preoperatively and postoperatively. (*A*) MRI T2 fast-spin echo (FSE)-FLAIR demonstrating significant peritumoral edema. (*B*) Diffusion sequence with significant hyperintensity commonly seen in higher grade meningiomas. (*C*) T1 fast spoiled gradient-echo (FSPGR) with contrast demonstrating the irregular outline of the meningioma and heterogeneous enhancement, consistent with higher grade meningioma (*D*) Postoperative MRI, T1 sequence with contrast after GTR.

reach statistical significance. Several reports have also found high MIB-1 labeling index correlates with recurrence,[16,17] although the Mayo group initially concluded that MIB-1 labeling was mainly useful for grading in borderline cases.

Another predictor of survival and recurrence for patients with aggressive meningiomas is age. The Central Brain Tumor Registry of the United States (CBTRUS) data suggests that age has one of the biggest effects on survival after diagnosis.

Table 1
World Health Organization classification for atypical and anaplastic meningiomas

Atypical meningioma	• 4–19 mitotic figures or 10 high-power fields OR
	• Brain invasion OR
	• Predominant choroid or clear cell morphology
	• 3 of the following histologic features
	  ○ Increased cellularity
	  ○ Small cells with high nuclear or cytoplasmic ratio
	  ○ Large and prominent nucleoli
	  ○ Patternless or sheet-like growth
	  ○ Foci of spontaneous or geographic necrosis

Anaplastic meningioma	• Excessive mitotic activity (>20 mitoses per 10 high-power fields) OR • Focal or diffuse loss of meningothelial differentiation at the light microscopic level resulting in sarcoma, carcinoma, or melanoma-like appearance OR • Predominant papillary or rhabdoid morphology

Data from Louis DN, Ohgaki H, Wiestler OD, et al. The 2007 WHO classification of tumours of the central nervous system. Acta Neuropathol 2007;114(2):97–109; and Sun SQ, Hawasli AH, Huang J, et al. An evidence-based treatment algorithm for the management of WHO grade II and III meningiomas. Neurosurg Focus 2015;38(3):E3.

Malignant meningiomas have a 10-year survival of 84.4% for patients 24 to 44 years old and 33.5% for patients older than 75 years.[2] Larger tumor size on presentation also predicts poor survival, mostly due to the tumor's ability to encompass neurovascular structures.[18] Overall outcomes with anaplastic meningiomas remain poor, with the average reported 5-year survival rates in the range of 30% to 60%.[1]

SURGICAL TREATMENT OPTIONS

Surgery is the main treatment of all types of meningiomas, allowing definitive histopathologic diagnosis and possible cure. The goals and technique of surgery in atypical and anaplastic meningiomas are essentially the same as for benign meningiomas. Whenever safely possible, Simpson grade I resection is attempted, with complete excision of the lesion along with a margin of healthy dura, as well as any affected bone. Atypical and anaplastic meningiomas often adhere to underlying cortex, making complete resection more challenging. Extent of resection appears to be the most important modifiable predictor of long-term outcome, with several studies showing clear benefit to GTR.[19]

Meningiomas, in general, are often highly vascular. Resection of large tumors with evidence of hypervascularity on preoperative imaging can sometimes be facilitated with embolization, especially when it is thought that the tumor's blood supply cannot be controlled early in surgery. This is usually accomplished using liquid embolic agents such as Onyx (ethylene vinyl-alcohol copolymer, ev3 Neurovascular, Irvine, CA, USA) but other methods and agents have been used. However, embolization carries its own set of risks, both from endovascular manipulation of the cerebral vasculature and from inadvertent occlusion of healthy branches by stray embolic agent. It is important to keep in mind that embolization is only worthwhile if it is thought that the combined risk of embolization and resection of the embolized tumor is less than the risk of up-front resection of the tumor.[20]

Like benign meningiomas, atypical and anaplastic meningiomas can usually be resected with relatively low risk of serious complications.[21] However, the morbidity and mortality are significantly lower when meningioma surgery is performed in a high-volume center while maintaining a maximal safe resection philosophy.[22] In a recent series of 45 atypical meningiomas, operated on a total of 62 times, including reoperations, postoperative complications were reported in 8 cases.[16] Only one of those complications was related to a reoperation. There were a total of 5 wound infections, one postoperative hematoma, one deep venous thrombosis, and one case of cerebrospinal fluid rhinorrhea.[16] The specific risk of venous thromboembolic complications was studied in a recent large series of meningiomas, 20% of which were either atypical or anaplastic. The investigators reported venous thromboembolic events in 7% of subjects, and identified weight and postoperative immobilization as the main risk factors. Histologic grade did not have an effect on the incidence of thromboembolic complications.[23]

Perioperative anticonvulsants are routinely used at many centers due to the potentially devastating effects that seizures can have in the postoperative period. However, in a meta-analysis comprising 19 studies and 698 subjects with meningiomas (most of which were benign), routine use of anticonvulsants in meningioma did not prove beneficial for prevention of both early and late postoperative seizures.[24] In patients who present with seizures preoperatively or develop seizures during the follow-up period, long-term antiepileptic treatment is usually required. At the authors' institution, levetiracetam is used as the first-line treatment and follow-up with an epileptologist for long-term care is arranged.

BRACHYTHERAPY

Implantation of radioactive seeds has been attempted in patients with recurrent atypical and anaplastic meningiomas. In one study, median survival of 8 years after implantation was achieved.[25] However, 27% of subjects developed wound breakdown, necessitating surgical intervention. Another 27% developed radiation necrosis, requiring reoperation in half. Despite this, brachytherapy offers a treatment option in tumors for which radiosurgery is not an option.

RADIOTHERAPY TREATMENT OPTIONS

The decision to use radiation for atypical meningiomas remains controversial because clear guidelines on the use of adjuvant treatments do not exist. Primarily, the decision to radiate these patients is governed by the extent of resection of the tumor. For patients who have STR or biopsy, adjuvant radiation treatment provides an improved progression-free survival as indicated by several studies.[26–32] Generally, the use of adjuvant fractionated external beam RT (EBRT) or stereotactic radiosurgery (SRS) after STR for both atypical and anaplastic meningiomas is accepted in the neurosurgical community due to the high recurrence rate after surgery alone (grade IC recommendation).[15] Current guidelines of the National Comprehensive Cancer Network recommend GTR alone for accessible tumors with adjuvant RT reserved for incomplete resections or recurrences for both atypical and WHO grade I meningiomas.[33] However, because of the increased risk for disease relapse in atypical meningiomas in up to 30% of cases, even after GTR, the management paradigm for these lesions recently has been contended.[30]

Treatment with RT after GTR for atypical meningiomas has been associated with improved local control at 5 years. In a recent systematic review by the authors, 5-year local control was improved by 11% for patients in the GTR plus RT group compared with the GTR group ($P = .057$).[34] Additionally, the recurrence rates were also significantly improved from 34% to 15% with the use of adjuvant RT ($P = .005$). Nevertheless, there was no improvement in overall survival for patients who received adjuvant RT and salvage RT after recurrence. **Table 2** demonstrates local recurrence rates for atypical meningiomas treated with GTR and GTR plus RT.[34] Typically, radiation treatment with EBRT is dosed at 54 to 60 Gy fractionated over 6 weeks; albeit, SRS can also be efficacious depending on the size and location of the lesion.

The most recent study evaluating RT in anaplastic meningiomas was done in 2010 and recommends radiotherapy after all surgical resections.[35] In this group, 63 subjects underwent surgery followed by radiation. The 2-, 5-, and 10-year overall survival was 82%, 61%, and 40%, respectively, and the progression-free survival was 80%, 57%, and 40%, respectively. Among the nearly 50% of subjects who recurred, there was a significant survival benefit to repeat surgery.

PHARMACOLOGIC TREATMENT OPTIONS

For treatment of refractory atypical and anaplastic meningiomas with aggressive pathologic features, pharmacologic treatment is occasionally necessary. Several clinical trials investigating the benefit of immunotherapeutic and hormonal agents have been performed with minimal benefit.[5] Because of failed previous chemotherapeutic agents, including hydroxyurea, a search for targeted therapies has ensued.[36–38] Several types of meningiomas have been found to demonstrate a high expression of certain molecular targets including platelet-derived growth factor (PDGF), epidermal growth factor (EGF), vascular endothelial growth factor (VEGF), insulin-like growth factor (IGF), and transforming growth factor-beta (TGF-β).[5,39] Although clinical trials investigating EGFR and PDGFR have been unfruitful, other targets such as VEGF have shown some early promise.[40–43] In a recent review by the authors, the use of bevacizumab for treatment refractory meningiomas resulted in a progression-free survival of 18 months (n = 44) based on a systematic review of 3 separate patient groups. Dosing for bevacizumab varies between 5 to 10 mg/kg per intravenous treatment.

Hormonal influences on meningioma growth have been well documented during periods of hormonal excess.[44,45] The correlation between immunohistochemistry for endocrine markers (progesterone and estrogen) and tumor progression has resulted in a search for hormonal pharmacotherapy. However, estrogen modulators have had little efficacy for meningiomas secondary to their low expression rate. In a recent study of treatment-refractory meningiomas, tamoxifen only demonstrated minimal responses in 3 out of 10 subjects.[46] Progesterone receptors, however, seem to be more abundant on cell surfaces of meningiomas. Therefore, a search for potential inhibitors ensued. Early studies using mifepristone (RU486), an antiprogesterone agent, have demonstrated some early promising results with radiographic regression in approximately 30% of subjects.[47,48] Nevertheless, larger studies by the Southwest Oncology Group failed to demonstrate any significant benefit of RU486 for treatment refractory meningiomas with nearly 90% disease progression despite treatment.[49] Growth hormone receptors also are nearly universal in meningiomas; therefore growth hormone antagonists may be able to inhibit tumor growth through IGF-1 modulation. Some partial treatment effects have been demonstrated after treatment with somatostatin or similar hormonal therapeutics.[49]

TREATMENT RESISTANCE OR COMPLICATIONS

For patients with disease progression or residual disease who receive radiation, clinicians must

Table 2			
Recurrence rates for atypical meningiomas treated initially with gross total resection or gross total resection plus radiotherapy			
	GTR	GTR + RT	*P* Value
Recurrence	33.7%	15.0%	.005
1 y local control	90.1%	97%	.09
5-y local control	55.1%	67.7%	.057
Overall survival	89.7%	89.4%	.95

monitor for treatment effect by evaluating for potential pseudoprogression or radiation necrosis. Post-treatment changes after radiation may occur for meningiomas depending on treatment type and time after radiation. Tumor swelling and suspected pseudoprogression in radiated meningiomas typically responds to corticosteroids within the first 6 months. Lesional progression 6 months after RT raises suspicion for radiation necrosis or true tumor progression. Patient with lesions suspicious for tumor progression or radiation necrosis should be serially monitored for radiographic changes or worsening symptoms. Patients who develop meningiomas refractory to both surgery and radiation continue to be very difficult to treat. For recurrent WHO II or III meningiomas, the progression-free survival at 6 months is only 29% and the treatment algorithm becomes more complex.[50] Repeat surgery for resection remains the best option in patients who can tolerate such an intervention.

Interestingly, an improved benefit was noted if the patient underwent a near total resection after tumor recurrence followed by radiotherapy versus a GTR followed by radiotherapy.[35] This suggests that attempts to achieve a GTR in these recurrent invasive meningiomas may sometimes be associated with increased risk. Therefore, the best philosophy is maximal safe resection on the first and second surgery.

Fig. 2 shows suggested treatment or management protocols for atypical and anaplastic meningiomas.

EXPERIMENTAL THERAPIES

Certain patients with treatment refractory meningiomas may be candidates for experimental therapies. Laser interstitial therapy (LITT) relies on stereotactic navigation-based catheter systems to induce thermal ablation of the target lesion.

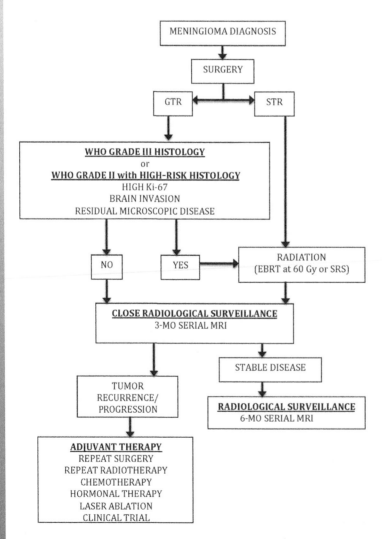

Fig. 2. Management paradigm for atypical and anaplastic meningiomas. (*Data from* Sun SQ, Hawasli AH, Huang J, et al. An evidence-based treatment algorithm for the management of WHO grade II and III meningiomas. Neurosurg Focus 2015;38(3):E3.)

For patients with multiple meningiomas, poor surgical candidates, or surgically inaccessible lesions, LITT may be an alternative option to cytoreductive surgery. Additional nonpharmacological options, including alternating electrical fields, may also be a theoretic option for highly aggressive meningiomas. Alternating electric fields interfere with cellular mitoses during anaphase through an external device that is calibrated to the tumor location. Another potential treatment of recurrent aggressive meningiomas with a high proliferative index is tumor treating field and is currently being investigated with a clinical trial. Finally, additional tumor markers continue to be isolated. For example, increased PD-L1 has been shown to increase expression on aggressive meningiomas and could lead to the use of checkpoint inhibitors.[51] These molecular targets are currently being investigated as potential targets for clinical trials.

EVALUATION OF OUTCOME AND LONG-TERM RECOMMENDATIONS

After treatment of atypical or anaplastic meningiomas, patients must be monitored very closely for disease progression. The Response Assessment in Neuro-Oncology (RANO) group criteria help monitor treatment response by measuring maximal cross-sectional area and clinical outcome after treatment. Responses are categorized as complete (disappearance of lesion), partial (>50% radiographic change), stable (<50% radiographic response), or progression (increase in size by 25%). Although the RANO criteria apply definitely to gliomas, using the RANO criteria for meningioma response may also help guide management protocols. Careful monitoring every 3 to 6 months with serial contrast-enhanced MRIs may be necessary depending on pathologic condition, proliferative index, extent of resection, and symptomatology.

SUMMARY AND DISCUSSION

Atypical and anaplastic meningiomas represent a small percentage of meningiomas. These lesions remain aggressive and difficult to treat. Surgery is the initial treatment option for both atypical and anaplastic meningiomas but recurrences remain more complex and difficult to treat. Over the past few decades, advances in surgical technique, radiation, and medical therapies have resulted in a modest improvement in overall survival; however, more prospective data are needed. A large number and variety of promising clinical trials have resulted from development of new minimally invasive techniques and targeted molecular therapies based on continuous research into these aggressive meningiomas.

REFERENCES

1. Hanft S, Canoll P, Bruce JN. A review of malignant meningiomas: diagnosis, characteristics, and treatment. J Neurooncol 2010;99(3):433–43.
2. Ostrom QT, Gittleman H, Liao P, et al. CBTRUS statistical report: primary brain and central nervous system tumors diagnosed in the United States in 2007-2011. Neuro Oncol 2014;16(Suppl 4):iv1–63.
3. Rogers L, Gilbert M, Vogelbaum M. Intracranial meningiomas of atypical (WHO grade II) histology. J Neurooncol 2010;99:393–405.
4. Moliterno J, Cope WP, Vartanian ED, et al. Survival in patients treated for anaplastic meningioma. J Neurosurg 2015;123(1):23–30.
5. Wen PY, Quant E, Drappatz J, et al. Medical therapies for meningiomas. J Neurooncol 2010;99(3):365–78.
6. Louis DN, Ohgaki H, Wiestler OD, et al. The 2007 WHO classification of tumours of the central nervous system. Acta Neuropathol 2007;114(2):97–109.
7. Alexiou GA, Gogou P, Markoula S, et al. Management of meningiomas. Clin Neurol Neurosurg 2010; 112(3):177–82.
8. Kane AJ, Sughrue ME, Rutkowski MJ, et al. Anatomic location is a risk factor for atypical and malignant meningiomas. Cancer 2011;117(6): 1272–8.
9. Modha A, Gutin PH. Diagnosis and treatment of atypical and anaplastic meningiomas: a review. Neurosurgery 2005;57(3):538–50 [discussion: 50].
10. Enokizono M, Morikawa M, Matsuo T, et al. The rim pattern of meningioma on 3D FLAIR imaging: correlation with tumor-brain adhesion and histological grading. Magn Reson Med Sci 2014;13(4):251–60.
11. Yue Q, Isobe T, Shibata Y, et al. New observations concerning the interpretation of magnetic resonance spectroscopy of meningioma. Eur Radiol 2008; 18(12):2901–11.
12. Cushing HW, Eisenhardt L. Meningiomas: Their Classification, Regional Behavior, Life History, and Surgical End Results. Springfield, Ill: Charles C Thomas; 1938. p. 47–50.
13. Cushing HW, Eisenhardt L. Meningiomas: Their Classification, Regional Behavior, Life History, and Surgical End Results. Springfield, Ill: Charles C Thomas; 1938. p. 669–719.
14. Perry A, Scheithauer BW, Stafford SL, et al. "Malignancy" in meningiomas: a clinicopathologic study of 116 patients, with grading implications. Cancer 1999;85(9):2046–56.
15. Sun SQ, Hawasli AH, Huang J, et al. An evidence-based treatment algorithm for the management of

WHO grade II and III meningiomas. Neurosurg Focus 2015;38(3):E3.

16. Klinger DR, Flores BC, Lewis JJ, et al. Atypical meningiomas: recurrence, reoperation, and radiotherapy. World Neurosurg 2015;84(3):839–45.

17. Bruna J, Brell M, Ferrer I, et al. Ki-67 proliferative index predicts clinical outcome in patients with atypical or anaplastic meningioma. Neuropathology 2007;27(2):114–20.

18. Ferraro DJ, Funk RK, Blackett JW, et al. A retrospective analysis of survival and prognostic factors after stereotactic radiosurgery for aggressive meningiomas. Radiat Oncol 2014;9:38.

19. Zhu H, Xie Q, Zhou Y, et al. Analysis of prognostic factors and treatment of anaplastic meningioma in China. J Clin Neurosci 2015;22(4):690–5.

20. Ashour R, Aziz-Sultan A. Preoperative tumor embolization. Neurosurg Clin N Am 2014;25(3):607–17.

21. Sughrue ME, Rutkowski MJ, Shangari G, et al. Risk factors for the development of serious medical complications after resection of meningiomas. Clinical article. J Neurosurg 2011;114(3):697–704.

22. Curry WT, McDermott MW, Carter BS, et al. Craniotomy for meningioma in the United States between 1988 and 2000: decreasing rate of mortality and the effect of provider caseload. J Neurosurg 2005; 102(6):977–86.

23. Hoefnagel D, Kwee LE, van Putten EH, et al. The incidence of postoperative thromboembolic complications following surgical resection of intracranial meningioma. A retrospective study of a large single center patient cohort. Clin Neurol Neurosurg 2014; 123:150–4.

24. Komotar RJ, Raper DM, Starke RM, et al. Prophylactic antiepileptic drug therapy in patients undergoing supratentorial meningioma resection: a systematic analysis of efficacy. J Neurosurg 2011; 115(3):483–90.

25. Ware ML, Larson DA, Sneed PK, et al. Surgical resection and permanent brachytherapy for recurrent atypical and malignant meningioma. Neurosurgery 2004;54(1):55–63 [discussion: 4].

26. Aizer AA, Arvold ND, Catalano P, et al. Adjuvant radiation therapy, local recurrence, and the need for salvage therapy in atypical meningioma. Neuro Oncol 2014;16(11):1547–53.

27. Lee KD, DePowell JJ, Air EL, et al. Atypical meningiomas: is postoperative radiotherapy indicated? Neurosurg Focus 2013;35(6):E15.

28. Hammouche S, Clark S, Wong AH, et al. Long-term survival analysis of atypical meningiomas: survival rates, prognostic factors, operative and radiotherapy treatment. Acta Neurochir (Wien) 2014; 156(8):1475–81.

29. Sun SQ, Cai C, Murphy RK, et al. Management of atypical cranial meningiomas, part 2: predictors of progression and the role of adjuvant radiation after

subtotal resection. Neurosurgery 2014;75(4):356–63 [discussion: 63].

30. Mair R, Morris K, Scott I, et al. Radiotherapy for atypical meningiomas. J Neurosurg 2011;115(4):811–9.

31. Park HJ, Kang HC, Kim IH, et al. The role of adjuvant radiotherapy in atypical meningioma. J Neurooncol 2013;115(2):241–7.

32. Jo K, Park HJ, Nam DH, et al. Treatment of atypical meningioma. J Clin Neurosci 2010;17(11):1362–6.

33. National Comprehensive Cancer System Network. Central nervous system cancers. J Natl Compr Canc Netw 2013;11(9):1114–51.

34. Hasan S, Young M, Albert T, et al. The role of adjuvant radiotherapy after gross total resection of atypical meningiomas. World Neurosurg 2015;83(5):808–15.

35. Sughrue ME, Sanai N, Shangari G, et al. Outcome and survival following primary and repeat surgery for World Health Organization Grade III meningiomas. J Neurosurg 2010;113(2):202–9.

36. Schrell UM, Rittig MG, Anders M, et al. Hydroxyurea for treatment of unresectable and recurrent meningiomas. I. Inhibition of primary human meningioma cells in culture and in meningioma transplants by induction of the apoptotic pathway. J Neurosurg 1997; 86(5):845–52.

37. Schrell UM, Rittig MG, Anders M, et al. Hydroxyurea for treatment of unresectable and recurrent meningiomas. II. Decrease in the size of meningiomas in patients treated with hydroxyurea. J Neurosurg 1997; 86(5):840–4.

38. Loven D, Hardoff R, Sever ZB, et al. Non-resectable slow-growing meningiomas treated by hydroxyurea. J Neurooncol 2004;67(1–2):221–6.

39. Smith JS, Lal A, Harmon-Smith M, et al. Association between absence of epidermal growth factor receptor immunoreactivity and poor prognosis in patients with atypical meningioma. J Neurosurg 2007;106(6):1034–40.

40. Norden AD, Raizer JJ, Abrey LE, et al. Phase II trials of erlotinib or gefitinib in patients with recurrent meningioma. J Neurooncol 2010;96(2):211–7.

41. Wen PY, Yung WK, Lamborn KR, et al. Phase II study of imatinib mesylate for recurrent meningiomas (North American Brain Tumor Consortium study 01-08). Neuro Oncol 2009;11(6):853–60.

42. Provias J, Claffey K, delAguila L, et al. Meningiomas: role of vascular endothelial growth factor/vascular permeability factor in angiogenesis and peritumoral edema. Neurosurgery 1997;40(5):1016–26.

43. Kaley TJ, Wen P, Schiff D, et al. Phase II trial of sunitinib for recurrent and progressive atypical and anaplastic meningioma. Neuro Oncol 2015;17(1):116–21.

44. Wahab M, Al-Azzawi F. Meningioma and hormonal influences. Climacteric 2003;6(4):285–92.

45. Kanaan I, Jallu A, Kanaan H. Management strategy for meningioma in pregnancy: a clinical study. Skull Base 2003;13(4):197–203.

46. Goodwin JW, Crowley J, Eyre HJ, et al. A phase II evaluation of tamoxifen in unresectable or refractory meningiomas: a Southwest Oncology Group study. J Neurooncol 1993;15(1):75–7.

47. Grunberg SM, Weiss MH, Spitz IM, et al. Treatment of unresectable meningiomas with the antiprogesterone agent mifepristone. J Neurosurg 1991;74(6): 861–6.

48. Lamberts SW, Tanghe HL, Avezaat CJ, et al. Mifepristone (RU 486) treatment of meningiomas. J Neurol Neurosurg Psychiatry 1992;55(6):486–90.

49. Norden AD, Drappatz J, Wen PY. Targeted drug therapy for meningiomas. Neurosurg Focus 2007; 23(4):E12.

50. Kaley T, Barani I, Chamberlain M, et al. Historical benchmarks for medical therapy trials in surgery- and radiation-refractory meningioma: a RANO review. Neuro Oncol 2014;16(6):829–40.

51. Du Z, Abedalthagafi M, Aizer AA, et al. Increased expression of the immune modulatory molecule PD-L1 (CD274) in anaplastic meningioma. Oncotarget 2015;6(7):4704–16.

Medical Management of Meningiomas

Current Status, Failed Treatments, and Promising Horizons

Michael Karsy, MD, PhD[a], Jian Guan, MD[a],
Adam Cohen, MD[b], Howard Colman, MD, PhD[a,b],
Randy L. Jensen, MD, PhD[a,b,c],*

KEYWORDS

- Targeted treatment • Meningiomas • Genetics • Medical management

KEY POINTS

- Meningiomas have the propensity for aggressive recurrence and resistance to traditional therapy.
- Only alpha-interferon, somatostatin receptor agonists, and vascular endothelial growth factor inhibitors are currently recommended for medical treatment of meningiomas.
- Novel therapeutic approaches and combinations may be a useful method in the treatment of aggressive meningiomas.

INTRODUCTION

Meningiomas are mostly benign tumors in adults that arise from the arachnoidal cap cells[1] intracranially and in the spine with an incidence of 7 44;100,000.[2] Most meningiomas are World Health Organization (WHO) grade I (80%); however, atypical grade II (15%–20%) and anaplastic grade III (1%–3%) tumors are relatively common and show a greater propensity for recurrence and therapeutic resistance.[3] Changes introduced in the 2007 WHO guidelines have led to an increase in the relative percentage of grade II and III meningiomas. Risk factors for meningioma include older age, a variety of genetic mutations and family disorders, ionizing radiation, head trauma, and sex.[1] Current therapeutic modalities include maximal safe gross total resection (GTR) followed by radiotherapy for higher-grade or recurrent lesions.[4] The Simpson grade, evaluating the degree of surgical resection, continues to be a viable tool for predicting survival and recurrence rates.[5] WHO grade II meningiomas show 5-year local control rates of 78% to 100% and 5-year progression-free survival (PFS) rates of 74% to 100% with GTR and radiotherapy.[6,7] WHO grade III meningiomas show 5-year PFS rates of 15% to 57% and 5-year overall survival (OS) of 47% to 61% with GTR and radiotherapy.[7] Although surgery and radiotherapy have been widely studied in the treatment and control of meningiomas, chemotherapeutic and targeted drugs have limited clinical efficacy.

The current National Comprehensive Cancer Network (NCCN) Clinical Practice Guidelines in Oncology (NCCN Guidelines, www.nccn.org) recommend radiological evaluation with biopsy if needed, as first-line steps in the evaluation of meningioma (**Fig. 1**). After radiographic or biopsy-proven diagnosis, asymptomatic meningiomas are recommended for surgery if they are accessible

[a] Department of Neurosurgery, Clinical Neurosciences Center, University of Utah, 175 N. Medical Drive East, Salt Lake City, UT 84132, USA; [b] Department of Oncological Sciences, Huntsman Cancer Institute, University of Utah, 2000 Circle of Hope, Salt Lake City, UT 84112, USA; [c] Department of Radiation Oncology, Huntsman Cancer Institute, University of Utah, 2000 Circle of Hope, Salt Lake City, UT 84112, USA
* Corresponding author. Departments of Neurosurgery, Radiation Oncology, and Oncological Sciences, Clinical Neuroscience Center, University of Utah, 175 North Medical Drive, Salt Lake City, UT 84132.
E-mail address: randy.jensen@hsc.utah.edu

Neurosurg Clin N Am 27 (2016) 249–260
http://dx.doi.org/10.1016/j.nec.2015.11.002
1042-3680/16/$ – see front matter © 2016 Elsevier Inc. All rights reserved.

A

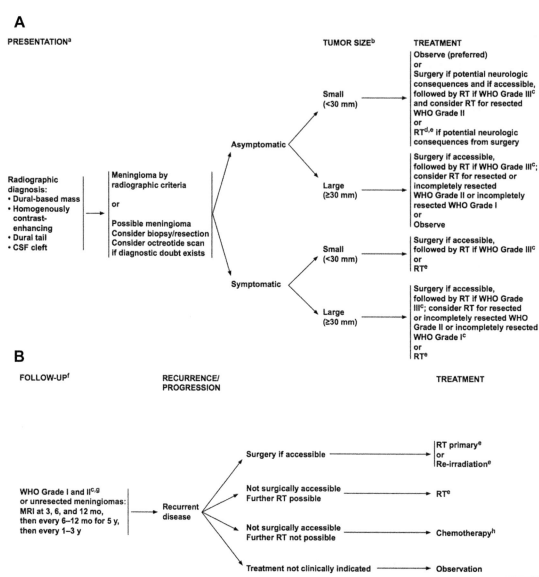

PRESENTATION[a]

Radiographic diagnosis:
• Dural-based mass
• Homogenously contrast-enhancing
• Dural tail
• CSF cleft

Meningioma by radiographic criteria

or

Possible meningioma
Consider biopsy/resection
Consider octreotide scan if diagnostic doubt exists

Asymptomatic

TUMOR SIZE[b]

Small (<30 mm)

Large (≥30 mm)

Symptomatic

Small (<30 mm)

Large (≥30 mm)

TREATMENT

Observe (preferred)
or
Surgery if potential neurologic consequences and if accessible, followed by RT if WHO Grade III[c] and consider RT for resected WHO Grade II
or
RT[d,e] if potential neurologic consequences from surgery

Surgery if accessible, followed by RT if WHO Grade III[c]; consider RT for resected or incompletely resected WHO Grade II or incompletely resected WHO Grade I
or
Observe

Surgery if accessible, followed by RT if WHO Grade III[c]
or
RT[e]

Surgery if accessible, followed by RT if WHO Grade III[c]; consider RT for resected or incompletely resected WHO Grade II or incompletely resected WHO Grade I[c]
or
RT[e]

B

FOLLOW-UP[f]

WHO Grade I and II[c,g] or unresected meningiomas:
MRI at 3, 6, and 12 mo, then every 6–12 mo for 5 y, then every 1–3 y

RECURRENCE/PROGRESSION

Recurrent disease

Surgery if accessible

Not surgically accessible
Further RT possible

Not surgically accessible
Further RT not possible

Treatment not clinically indicated

TREATMENT

RT primary[e]
or
Re-irradiation[e]

RT[e]

Chemotherapy[h]

Observation

Fig. 1. NCCN guidelines version 1.2015: meningiomas. (*A*) Guidelines for the treatment of newly diagnosed meningioma. For small, asymptomatic lesions, observation is generally recommended after clinical and radiographic evaluation. For larger asymptomatic lesions, surgical resection is typically recommended, particularly when they are located in more accessible areas or there are potential neurologic consequences to a conservative approach. Depending on tumor grade, subsequent radiotherapy (RT) may also be recommended. Tumors that are symptomatic are referred for surgical resection when feasible. These patients are monitored closely after surgery and may undergo RT depending on tumor grade and level of resection. CSF, cerebrospinal fluid. (*B*) Guidelines for the treatment of recurrent meningioma. After treatment, patients are followed at 3, 6, and 12 months with contrast-enhanced MRI. After 1 year, the MRIs are repeated every 6 to 12 months for 5 years and then every 1 to 3 years. The management of recurrence depends on individual factors, personalized to the patient. For instance, surgical treatment followed by RT may be used if the recurrence is accessible, whereas RT or chemotherapy, or observation, may be recommended if the lesion is surgically inaccessible. [a] Multidisciplinary input for treatment planning if feasible. [b] The median growth rate for meningiomas is 4 mm per annum. [c] WHO Grade I = benign meningioma; WHO Grade II = atypical meningioma; WHO Grade III = malignant (anaplastic) meningioma. [d] RT can be either external-beam or stereotactic radiosurgery (SRS). [e] Principles of brain tumor radiation therapy: WHO grade I meningiomas may be treated by fractionated conformal radiotherapy with doses of 45 to 54 Gy. For WHO grade II meningiomas undergoing radiation, treatment should be directed to gross tumor (if present) and surgical bed + a margin (1–2 cm) to a dose of 54 to 60 Gy in 1.8 to 2.0 Gy fractions. Consider limiting margin expansion into the brain parenchyma if there is no evidence of brain invasion. WHO grade III meningiomas should be treated as malignant tumors with treatment directed to gross tumor (if present) and surgical and large (≥30 mm) or there is a concern regarding a potential neurologic consequence but can otherwise be observed. Surgery is also recommended for lesions that are symptomatic and accessible at any size or stage. After surgery, radiotherapy is recommended as a standard for WHO grade III lesions but is optional for WHO grade I or II lesions. For low-grade lesions, follow-up with MRI is recommended at 3, 6, and 12 months, then every 6 to 12 months for another 5 years, and less frequently beyond 5 years. Higher-grade lesions are monitored more closely. For recurrent meningiomas not amenable to surgery or radiation therapy, the current NCCN Guidelines recommend only 3 classes of chemotherapeutic agents as medical treatments in meningiomas because clinical trials have shown partial benefits.[8–10] These agents include α-interferon, somatostatin receptor agonists, and vascular endothelial growth factor (VEGF) inhibitors.

The focus of the recent prospective RTOG 0539 trial, which has closed enrollment, is to evaluate the best current care for meningiomas (www. rtog.org). Patients were categorized into groups based on the risk of recurrence, and PFS will be assessed at 3 years. The low-risk group includes patients with Simpson grade I–III resections or Simpson grade IV–V resections and grade I tumor; these patients are observed after surgical treatment. The intermediate group includes patients with WHO grade II or recurrent WHO grade I lesions that are treated with planned conformal radiotherapy or intensity-modulated radiotherapy (IMRT; 54 Gy in 30 fractions). The high-risk group includes patients with WHO grade III or recurrent WHO grade II tumors who were treated with planned IMRT (60 Gy in 30 fractions). The results of this prospective study will aid in elucidating the therapeutic efficacy of various treatment approaches. Furthermore, the use of medical treatments can be compared as additive treatments to these approaches.

A recent meta-analysis of 47 publications evaluating various treatment options in meningioma concluded that significant heterogeneity of inclusion and response criteria made evaluation of effective treatments more challenging[11] but suggested that PFS-6 was easily extractable from most studies and could be compared across treatment types. For WHO I meningiomas, the weighted average PFS-6 was 29%, whereas the average for WHO II/III meningiomas was 26%. Furthermore, this analysis indicated that a PFS-6 of greater than 40% for grade I meningiomas and greater than 30% for grade II/III meningiomas would reasonably suggest that a treatment had therapeutic efficacy. These results provide a starting point for powering studies and evaluating clinically meaningful impacts of diverse treatment options.

In this review, various medical therapies that have been evaluated in meningiomas (**Table 1**) are discussed. Many of these agents have had limited success, with results hindered by small study sizes and heterogenous inclusion criteria. Despite these limitations, previous trials have helped in the ongoing design of the next generation of clinical trials and combination therapies to improve on meningoma treatment.

MUTATIONS IN MENINGIOMA

Many recent studies have helped define the mutational background of meningiomas, aiding in understanding the pathophysiology of meningiomas and suggesting new therapeutic targets. Deletion of neurofibromin 2 (*NF2*, also known as Merlin and moesin-, ezrin-, radixin [ERM]-like protein), which is found on chromosome 22q12, is a well-characterized mutation in sporadic meningioma found in upwards of 50% to 60% of patients.[12] The NF2 protein is a member of the 4.1 ERM family of proteins localized to the cell membrane and involved in regulating cytoskeletal proteins (eg, paxillin, actin, syntenin) involved in actin cytoskeletal organization, cell–cell adhesion, and migration.[1,13] Loss of chromosome 22 is also common, occurring in 54% to 78% of sporadic meningiomas.[12] Merlin has been shown to play a key role in regulating meningioma cell proliferation and tumor formation in mouse models as well as in regulating multiple downstream pathways.[14] Other

---

bed + a margin (2–3 cm) receiving 59.4 to 60 Gy in 1.8 to 2.0 Gy fractions. WHO grade I meningiomas may also be treated with SRS doses of 12 to 16 Gy in a single fraction when appropriate. [f] Less frequent follow-up after 5 to 10 years. [g] More frequent imaging may be required for WHO grade III meningiomas and for meningiomas of any grade that are treated for recurrence or with chemotherapy. [h] Interferon-α (category 2B), somatostatin analogue (if octreotide scan positive), sunitinib (category 2B). (*Adapted from* the NCCN Clinical Practice Guidelines in Oncology (NCCN Guidelines®) for Central Nervous System Cancers V.1.2015. © 2015 National Comprehensive Cancer Network, Inc. The NCCN Guidelines® and illustrations herein may not be reproduced in any form for any purpose without the express written permission of the NCCN. To view the most recent and complete version of the NCCN Guidelines, go online to NCCN.org. NATIONAL COMPREHENSIVE CANCER NETWORK®, NCCN®, NCCN GUIDELINES®, and all other NCCN Contents are trademarks owned by the National Comprehensive Cancer Network, Inc.)

Table 1
Summary of studies evaluating medical treatments in meningiomas

Reference	Agent	Mechanism	n	WHO Grade				Median PFS	PFS-6
				N/A	I	II	III		
Kim et al,[62] 2012	Hydroxyurea	Ribonucleotide reductase inhibitor	—	—	—	—	—	—	—
Schrell et al,[52] 1997	Hydroxyurea	Ribonucleotide reductase inhibitor	4	—	3	—	—	—	—
Newton et al,[53] 2000	Hydroxyurea	Ribonucleotide reductase inhibitor	17	—	16	3	1	80 wk	—
Mason et al,[54] 2002	Hydroxyurea	Ribonucleotide reductase inhibitor	20	—	16	3	1	—	—
Rosenthal et al,[55] 2002	Hydroxyurea	Ribonucleotide reductase inhibitor	15	—	10	5	—	—	—
Loven et al,[56] 2004	Hydroxyurea	Ribonucleotide reductase inhibitor	12	—	8	4	—	13 mo	—
Hahn et al,[57] 2005	Hydroxyurea with radiotherapy		21	4	13	2	2	—	—
Weston et al,[58] 2006	Hydroxyurea	Ribonucleotide reductase inhibitor	6	1	5	—	—	—	—
Chamberlain & Johnston,[59] 2011	Hydroxyurea	Ribonucleotide reductase inhibitor	60	—	60	—	—	4 mo	10%
Chamberlain,[60] 2012	Hydroxyurea	Ribonucleotide reductase inhibitor	35	—	—	22	13	2 mo	3%
Chamberlain et al,[79] 2004	Temozolomide	Alkylating agent	16	—	16	—	—	5 mo	0%
Chamberlain et al,[80] 2006	Irinotecan	Topoisomerase 1 inhibitor	16	—	16	—	—	4.5 m	6%
Chamberlain,[78] 1996	Cyclophosphamide + Adriamycin (doxorubicin) + vincristine (CAV)	Cytotoxic chemotherapy	14	—	—	—	14	4.6 y	—
Kaba et al,[91] 1997	Interferon-α	Immunomodulation	6	—	2	1	3	—	—
Muhr et al,[92] 2001	Interferon-α	Immunomodulation	12	2	6	1	3	—	—
Chamberlain & Glantz,[10] 2008	Interferon-α	Immunomodulation	35	—	35	—	—	7 mo	54%
Lamberts et al,[72] 1992	Mifepristone (RU486)	Antiprogesterone	12	—	—	—	—	—	—
Grunberg et al,[69] 1991	Mifepristone (RU486)	Antiprogesterone	14	2	7	3	2	—	—
Grunberg et al,[70] 2006	Mifepristone (RU486)	Antiprogesterone	28	4	22	—	2	—	—
Touat et al,[71] 2014	Mifepristone (RU486)	Antiprogesterone	3	—	3	—	—	—	—
de Keizer & Smit,[73] 2004	Mifepristone (RU486)	Antiprogesterone	2	—	—	—	—	—	—

Study	Agent	Mechanism							
Grunberg & Weiss,[67] 1990	Megestrol acetate	Progesterone receptor agonist	9	—	8	—	1	—	—
Jaaskelainen et al,[68] 1986	Medroxy-progesterone acetate	Synthetic progesterone	5	—	4	—	1	—	—
Markwalder et al,[75] 1985	Tamoxifen	Antiestrogen	6	—	—	—	—	—	—
Goodwin et al,[76] 1993	Tamoxifen	Antiestrogen	21	—	—	—	—	15.1 mo	—
Runzi et al,[84] 1989	Octreotide	Somatostatin analogue	1	1	—	—	—	—	—
Garcia-Luna et al,[85] 1993	Octreotide	Somatostatin analogue	3	—	2	—	1	—	—
Jaffrain-Rea et al,[86] 1998	Octreotide	Somatostatin analogue	1	—	—	—	—	—	—
Johnson et al,[87] 2011	Octreotide	Somatostatin analogue	11	—	3	3	5	17 wk	—
Chamberlain et al,[8] 2007	Sandostatin LAR	Somatostatin analogue	16	—	8	3	3	5 mo	44%
Norden et al,[89] 2015	Pasireotide LAR	Somatostatin analogue	26	—	9	17	—	20 wk	29%
Simo et al,[88] 2014	Octreotide	Somatostatin analogue	9	—	—	5	4	4.23 mo	44%
Wen et al,[49] 2009	Imatinib	PDGFR TKI	23	—	12	5	5	2 mo	29.40%
Raizer et al,[50] 2010	Erlotinib	EGFR TKI	1	—	—	1	—	—	—
Norden et al,[51] 2010	Erlotinib or gefitinib	EGFR TKI	25	—	8	9	8	10 wk	28%
Reardon et al,[61] 2012	Imatinib and hydroxyurea	PDGFR TKI + ribonucleotide reductase inhibitor	21	—	8	9	4	7 mo	61.90%
Raizer et al,[50] 2010	Vatalanib (PTL-787)	VEGFR + PDGFR TKI	21	—	—	14	7	—	37.50%
Raizer et al,[48] 2014	Vatalanib (PTL-787)	VEGFR + PDGFR TKI	25	—	2	14	8	6.5 mo	37.50%
Kaley et al,[9] 2015	Sunitinib	VEGFR + PDGFR TKI	36	—	—	30	6	5.2 mo	42%
Puchner et al,[41] 2010	Bevacizumab	Anti-VEGFR antibody	1	—	—	—	1	—	—
Goutagny et al,[42] 2011	Bevacizumab	Anti-VEGFR antibody	1	1	—	—	—	—	—
Wilson & Heth,[43] 2012	Bevacizumab + paclitaxel	Anti-VEGFR antibody	1	—	1	—	—	15 mo	—
Lou et al,[44] 2012	Bevacizumab	Anti-VEGFR antibody	14	1	5	5	3	17.9 mo	85.70%
Nayak et al,[45] 2012	Bevacizumab	Anti-VEGFR antibody	15	—	—	6	9	26 wk	43.80%
Nunes et al,[47] 2013	Bevacizumab	Anti-VEGFR antibody	15	—	—	—	—	15 mo	—

Adapted from Kaley T, Barani I, Chamberlain M, et al. Historical benchmarks for medical therapy trials in surgery- and radiation-refractory meningioma: a RANO review. Neuro Oncol 2014;16:830–1; with permission of Oxford University Press and the Society for Neuro-Oncology.

genes mutated with chromosome 22 loss include BAM22,[15] which is involved in intracellular transport of proteins in the Golgi network; INI1,[16] which is involved in chromatin remodeling; BCR (breakpoint cluster region); and TIMP-1.[17] Another mutated gene in the 4.1 ERM protein family, DAL-1, is involved in tumor progression rather than initiation and regulates multiple downstream molecules including JNK (c-Jun N-terminal kinase[18]) and 14-3-3 protein.[17] Other chromosomal abnormalities in meningioma include losses on 1p, 6q, 9p, 10, 14q, 18q, 19, and 20 as well as gains on 1q, 9q, 12q, 15q, 17q, and 20q with multiple involved genes.[12] The key signaling pathways and molecular signatures of meningiomas have yet to be fully developed.

Several key signaling pathways regulating cell proliferation and growth can be altered in meningiomas and a variety of other tumors. Activation of phosphatidylinositol 3-kinase (PI3K)/Akt pathway, through loss-of-function mutations or deletion of PTEN (phosphatase and tensin homolog) or through activating mutations in PIK3CA or AKT, can result in activation of mammalian target of rapamycin (mTOR) and is commonly seen in meningiomas.[19] Akt (AKT1) activation is more common in atypical and anaplastic meningioma. Mutation of AKT1 has been observed in a subset of NF2-mutated meningiomas associated with higher-grade tumors.[20] Targeting of PI3K/Akt/mTOR has been widely investigated in glioma but has not been extensively evaluated in meningioma.[21] Genes for upstream tyrosine kinases, including platelet-derived growth factor receptor-β (PDGFRβ), epidermal growth factor receptor (EGFR), and transforming growth factor (TGF), are commonly mutated in meningioma, can drive downstream pathways such as mTOR, and have been explored as targets.[22] These signaling pathways can act through a variety of downstream pathways including mitogen-activated protein kinase (MAPK) and phospholipase C.[19] MAPK and its associated signaling pathways have been targeted in a variety of cancers but have yet to be fully explored in meningioma treatment.[23] Transforming growth factor-β receptor (TGF-βR), a potent suppressor of tumor growth via the TGF signaling pathway, is lost in increasingly more aggressive grades of meningiomas.[24]

A variety of other mutations with potential roles as targets can be seen in meningiomas. Mutation of the reverse transcriptase subunit hTERT, which is involved in telomerase activity, is rare in grade I meningiomas (3%–21%) but common in atypical (58%–92%) and anaplastic meningiomas (100%).[1] Targeting of telomerases is an exciting area of research in regulating cancer senescence

and may have potential in treating meningiomas.[25] Cell-cycle–regulating proteins, such as p14ARF, p16INK4a (CDKN2A), and p15 (CDKN2B), are commonly described mutations in meningiomas with potential effects on aberrant cell proliferation.[26] Approaches in targeting cell-cycle regulators are forthcoming but limited clinically.[27] Alterations in hedgehog[28] and Notch pathway[29] signaling are also seen in meningiomas. Loss of E-cadherin involved in Wingless (WNT)/β-catenin signaling can be seen in 30% of meningiomas and correlates with more aggressive meningiomas.[17,30] Recent genomic studies have helped identify 4 key genes in non-NF2-mutated meningiomas: TRAF7 (tumor necrosis factor [TNF] receptor-associated factor 7), KLF-4 (Kruppel-like factor 4), AKT1, and SMO (smoothened), which are associated with more benign grades, chromosomal stability, and medial skull base locations.[31] Alternative methods of meningioma regulation have been seen in the impact of microRNA molecules (miRs), small nucleotide sequences involved in suppression of mRNA translation. Importantly, inducing or suppressing these molecules has been considered among the approaches in the treatment of tumors. Several miRs involved in regulating meningioma proliferation include miR-200a[32] and miR-224.[33] One study showed dysregulation of 13 miRs in benign meningiomas and 52 miRs in anaplastic meningioma.[34] These molecules target genes involved in regulating epithelial-mesenchymal transition, WNT, TGF-β, and VEGF.

ANGIOGENIC PATHWAY INHIBITORS

Expression of VEGF A can be seen in 79% of meningiomas and correlates with microvascular density and increased tumor grade.[35–37] Expression of hypoxia-inducible factor-1, a significant regulator of VEGF expression and hypoxia regulation, is also commonly seen in meningiomas.[38] Reductions in peritumoral edema and radiation necrosis have also been seen with VEGF inhibitors, suggesting a potential role of antiangiogenesis inhibitors as targeted therapy in meningioma.[39,40]

The efficacy of the VEGF-targeting agent bevacizumab in meningioma has been evaluated in several studies. Studies with bevacizumab have reported median PFS of 26 weeks to 17.9 months and PFS-6 of 37.5% to 85.7%.[11,41–45] Unfortunately, these studies are all retrospective, with populations that varied in grade, prior treatments, concomitant treatments, and percentage of patients with germ-line NF2 mutations. A recent study of 10 patients with meningioma and concurrent vestibular schwannomas (6 with NF2 mutation, 4 with recurrent meningioma) showed stable to improved disease in 8 patients with minor toxicity.[46] Another retrospective study of 15 patients with NF2 mutation harboring meningiomas and vestibular schwannomas showed decreased tumor size in 3 patients, which was nonsustained, with a median duration of response of less than 4 months.[47] A novel VEGF inhibitor, PTK787 (vatalanib), was evaluated in a prospective single-arm trial of 24 patients with meningioma; a PFS-6 of 37.5% for patients with grade III meningioma and 64.3% for patients with grade II meningiomas.[48] The combination VEGF/PDGFR inhibitor sunitinib was also evaluated in a prospective phase 2 trial in grade II–III meningiomas; the results indicated a PFS-6 of 42%.[11,48] Thus, small molecule inhibitors of VEGF and/or PDGF are the most promising systemic treatment for high-grade meningiomas, pending phase 3 trials.

TYROSINE KINASE RECEPTOR INHIBITORS

Targeting tyrosine kinase inhibitors (TRKIs), including imatinib (targeting PDGFR)[49] and erlotinib[50,51] and gefitinib[51] (both targeting EGFR), has been tried with minimal success in meningiomas. PFS-6 for TRKIs ranged from 28% to 44% and median PFS from 8 weeks to 5 months in prospective studies. Imatinib was evaluated in the North American Brain Tumor Consortium (NABTC) study 01-08 in a group of 22 individuals with recurrent grade I and II meningiomas.[49] The results suggested that imatinib was well tolerated, but median PFS was only 2 months and PFS-6 was 29.4%. Furthermore, tumor progression was more advanced in patients with malignant histologic features. In a pooled analysis of 2 NABTC prospective trials of EGFR inhibitors in meningiomas, 25 individuals with recurrent meningioma were treated with gefitinib (n = 16) or erlotinib (n = 9).[51] This study showed PFS-6 and OS-12 of 25% and 50% for benign tumors and 29% and 65% for grade II–III tumors, respectively. These results suggested that EGFR inhibitors did not show an appreciable impact on PFS as monotherapy.

HYDROXYUREA

Hydroxyurea has been widely studied in the treatment of meningioma, grades I through III. It was initially developed as a ribonucleotide reductase inhibitor inhibiting cell cycle for the treatment of myeloproliferative diseases and chronic myelogenous leukemia.[4] In meningioma, hydroxyurea has shown a range in median PFS of 10 to 80 weeks and PFS-6 of 3% to 10%.[52–61] These studies are limited by their retrospective design and small sample sizes. The use of concomitant therapies also complicates assessments of the efficacy of hydroxyurea. A recent retrospective study of 60 patients treated with hydroxyurea showed disease progression in 65% of patients, with a median PFS of 4 months.[59] Another retrospective study of 13 patients with WHO I and II meningioma treated with hydroxyurea showed stable disease in 10 patients with a median time to progression of 72.4 months.[62] Another recent study of 60 patients treated with hydroxyurea showed disease progression in 65% of patients, with a median PFS of 4 months.[59] In several studies, treatment with hydroxyurea has been combined with radiotherapy[57] or calcium channel blockers.[63–65] Although this combined treatment may be promising, a recent prospective trial from the authors' institution showed limited patient clinical and radiographic responsiveness to hydroxyurea, with a median PFS of 8 months and PFS-6 of 85% (Karsy et al., in press).

HORMONE RECEPTOR TARGETED AGENTS

The incidence of meningiomas in women has been shown to be twice as high as that in men, suggesting a hormonal influence on tumor pathogenesis.[1] Evaluation of meningiomas has shown a significant level of progesterone receptors but limited expression of estrogen receptors.[66] Several studies have evaluated the role of hormone receptor targeting agents in the treatment of meningioma. In an initial evaluation of megestrol in a series of 9 patients with meningiomas (8 grade I, 1 grade III), stable radiographic disease was described, but neither PFS nor long-term outcome was reported.[67] Medroxyprogesterone acetate, another synthetic progesterone receptor targeting agent, was also evaluated in a series of 5 meningiomas with limited results.[68] Mifepristone, a hormone receptor targeting agent with affinity for progesterone receptors, has been evaluated in several studies with mixed results.[69–73] Initially, evaluation of mifepristone in a series of 13 patients showed tumor regression in 5 of 13 patients and tolerance of drug therapy over 2 years; however, a recent systematic review found little evidence for an improvement in PFS.[69,74] Moreover, a randomized phase 3 trial of mifepristone in meningiomas was reported at the American Society of Clinical Oncology annual meeting in 2001 with negative results but has never been fully published. The findings of limited efficacy of mifepristone may be due to its evaluation in heterogeneous cohorts of patients as well as to variations in hormone receptors expressed.[74] Furthermore, mifepristone has shown a variety of non-hormone receptor-mediated effects on cell migration and apoptosis, suggesting additional roles for the agent. Tamoxifen, a selective estrogen receptor modulator used in the treatment of estrogen-receptor-positive breast cancer, was evaluated in several studies of patients with meningiomas.[75,76] A retrospective series of 21 patients with meningioma treated with tamoxifen showed response in only 1 patient and disease progression in 10 patients at 31-month follow-up.[76] Interestingly, a population study of patients treated with tamoxifen for breast cancer involving 227,535 women showed these women had a lower incidence of meningioma formation compared with women with breast cancer not treated with tamoxifen; the benefit persisted during 10 years of follow-up.[77]

CHEMOTHERAPEUTIC AGENTS

Another avenue of investigation has considered treatment of meningiomas with traditional cytotoxic chemotherapeutic agents. Use of combined cyclophosphamide, Adriamycin (doxorubicin), and vincristine (CAV therapy) after surgery and radiation as initial treatment of grade III meningioma was evaluated in a small cohort of 14 patients, demonstrating a median PFS of 4.6 years, PFS-6 of 6%, and radiographically stable disease in 12 of 14 patients.[78] Another approach evaluated the alkylating agent temozolomide in a phase II trial of 16 patients with refractory meningioma; this protocol showed no radiographic response and an unimpressive median PFS of 5 months.[79] The topoisomerase inhibitor irinotecan was ineffective in a series of 16 patients with median PFS of 4.5 months and PFS-6 of 6%[80]; however, evaluation of irinotecan in vitro and in vivo showed efficacy during treatment of meningioma.[81] Another agent that has been evaluated on a limited basis is the DNA-binding agent trabectedin, which inhibits transcription factor binding. It was found to inhibit meningioma in vivo but had limited efficacy in human treatment.[82] A recent in vitro evaluation of multiple chemotherapeutic agents (ie, carmustine, lomustine, cisplatin, daunorubicin, dacarbazine, paclitaxel, temozolomide, topotecan, vincristine, and etoposide) in 29 patient samples showed limited effective concentration required to reduce cell viability by 50%.[83] These results suggest that simple targeting with increasingly toxic doses of chemotherapeutic agents may not be effective in meningiomas and instead combination or alternative approaches may be necessary.

SOMATOSTATIN ANALOGUES

Somatostatin analogues, including octreotide, Sandostatin LAR, and pasireotide, have been evaluated in the treatment of meningioma.[8,84–89] Somatostatin, also known as growth hormone–inhibiting hormone, is secreted by the ventromedial nucleus of the hypothalamus and inhibits multiple pituitary, gastrointestinal, and pancreatic hormones. Meningiomas have been known to highly express somatostatin receptors.[8] One study evaluated 16 patients with recurrent meningioma treated with long-acting octreotide (Sandostatin LAR) and showed a median PFS of 5 months, PFS-6 of 44%, and median OS of 7.5 months.[8] Furthermore, one-third of patients showed stable disease after treatment. A recent trial in 34 patients of pasireotide LAR treatment in recurrent meningiomas with malignant histology showed a PFS-6 of 17% and median PFS of 15 weeks.[89] Furthermore, expression of somatostatin receptor 3 but not octreotide uptake or insulinlike growth factor-1 (IGF-1) levels was predictive of favorable response. The single-arm design of this trial precludes conclusions about whether somatostatin receptor expression is predictive or merely prognostic as a biomarker. A recent study of 9 patients with grade II and III meningioma treated with octreotide showed PFS-6 of 44.4%.[88] Combined treatment of octreotide, a somatostatin analogue, with everolimus, an mTOR inhibitor, has been evaluated during in vitro treatment of meningiomas.[90] Octreotide suppressed AKT activation during everolimus treatment and synergistically reduced expression of downstream proteins (ie, 4EBP1, p27, and cyclin D1).

IMMUNOMODULATION

Several studies have shown that treatment of meningioma with interferon-α has a therapeutic effect.[10,91,92] Interferon-α binds to the interferon-α/β receptor and is involved in cell resistance to viral infection but has been investigated as a cancer adjuvant therapy. The most recent study evaluated interferon-α in 35 cases of refractory grade I meningioma after standard therapies and showed a PFS-6 of 17%, suggesting limited activity.[93]

EMERGING APPROACHES

Several newer approaches in the treatment of meningioma have sought novel therapeutic targets. One strategy involved targeting meningiomas with growth hormone receptor antagonists because of their high expression of growth hormone receptors.[94] In vitro targeting with growth hormone antagonists can inhibit meningioma cell proliferation.[94] Furthermore, targeting of growth hormone receptors with pegvisomant via an in vivo flank model was shown to significantly reduce tumor volume, serum IGF-1 tissue concentration, and circulating IGFBP-3 (IGF binding protein 3) levels, but did not alter tumor tissue IGF-1 levels.[95] These results suggested inhibition of host tissue IGF-1 levels was able to reduce tumor proliferation. Another targeted approach involved the use of valproic acid to inhibit meningioma stem cells' function in vitro.[96] Valproic acid improved radiosensitivity and expression of apoptotic markers (eg, pH2AX, caspase-3, PARP) and decreased expression of stem cell markers (eg, Oct4). Another novel approach involved the use of TNF-related apoptosis-inducing ligand (TRAIL) in combination with bortezomib.[97] TRAIL, a cytokine that binds to death receptors DR4 (TRAIL-R1) and DR5 (TRAIL-R2) to induce apoptosis, and bortezomib, a proteosome inhibitor, synergistically inhibited meningioma cells in vitro. Bortezomib enhanced expression of TRAIL-R1 and TRAIL-R2 to allow ligand binding and apoptosis induction. Last, another recent study evaluated the role of 5-aminolevulinic acid (5-ALA) as a photosensitizing agent in meningioma treatment.[98] This group used 5-ALA during in vitro treatment of primary meningiomas and showed a significant, dose-dependent reduction in cell viability with a medial lethal dose between 25 and 50 µg/mL. These studies suggest a variety of targets as well as strategies, such as radiosensitizing agents, that warrant further investigation. PD-1 (programmed cell death 1) and PD-L1 (programmed death ligand 1), a receptor-ligand pairing that functions in the immune response to neoplasia, has been a successful target for various tumor types.[99,100] There have been no clinical trials to date investigating the PD-1/PD-L1 pathway inhibition in meningiomas, although recent studies demonstrating upregulated PD-L1 expression in anaplastic meningiomas suggest that such therapies have an impact.[101]

Among the limitations to the various approaches of targeting meningiomas have been the heterogenous patient samples and validation methods. Future prospective studies, such as the RTOG 0539 trial, will help to support current practice methods and identify standards of care and may ultimately serve as a basis for additional medical therapies. The use of prospective patient registries may also be a strategy to combine many of these smaller trials and achieve meaningful sample sizes for analysis.

REFERENCES

1. Choy W, Kim W, Nagasawa D, et al. The molecular genetics and tumor pathogenesis of meningiomas and the future directions of meningioma treatments. Neurosurg Focus 2011;30(5):E6.

2. Ostrom QT, Gittleman H, Farah P, et al. CBTRUS statistical report: primary brain and central nervous system tumors diagnosed in the United States in 2006-2010. Neuro Oncol 2013;15(Suppl 2):ii1–56.

3. Smith SJ, Boddu S, Macarthur DC. Atypical meningiomas: WHO moved the goalposts? Br J Neurosurg 2007;21(6):588–92.

4. Moazzam AA, Wagle N, Zada G. Recent developments in chemotherapy for meningiomas: a review. Neurosurg Focus 2013;35(6):E18.

5. Simpson D. The recurrence of intracranial meningiomas after surgical treatment. J Neurol Neurosurg Psychiatry 1957;20(1):22–39.

6. Hasan S, Young M, Albert T, et al. The role of adjuvant radiotherapy after gross total resection of atypical meningiomas. World Neurosurg 2015;83(5):808–15.

7. Sun SQ, Hawasli AH, Huang J, et al. An evidence-based treatment algorithm for the management of WHO grade II and III meningiomas. Neurosurg Focus 2015;38(3):E3.

8. Chamberlain MC, Glantz MJ, Fadul CE. Recurrent meningioma: salvage therapy with long-acting somatostatin analogue. Neurology 2007;69(10):969–73.

9. Kaley TJ, Wen P, Schiff D, et al. Phase II trial of sunitinib for recurrent and progressive atypical and anaplastic meningioma. Neuro Oncol 2015;17(1):116–21.

10. Chamberlain MC, Glantz MJ. Interferon-alpha for recurrent World Health Organization grade 1 intracranial meningiomas. Cancer 2008;113(8):2146–51.

11. Kaley T, Barani I, Chamberlain M, et al. Historical benchmarks for medical therapy trials in surgery and radiation-refractory meningioma: a RANO review. Neuro Oncol 2014;16(6):829–40.

12. Ragel BT, Jensen RL. Molecular genetics of meningiomas. Neurosurg Focus 2005;19(5):E9.

13. Xu HM, Gutmann DH. Merlin differentially associates with the microtubule and actin cytoskeleton. J Neurosci Res 1998;51(3):403–15.

14. Stamenkovic I, Yu Q. Merlin, a "magic" linker between extracellular cues and intracellular signaling pathways that regulate cell motility, proliferation, and survival. Curr Protein Pept Sci 2010;11(6):471–84.

15. Peyrard M, Fransson I, Xie YG, et al. Characterization of a new member of the human beta-adaptin gene family from chromosome 22q12, a candidate meningioma gene. Hum Mol Genet 1994;3(8):1393–9.

16. Schmitz U, Mueller W, Weber M, et al. INI1 mutations in meningiomas at a potential hotspot in exon 9. Br J Cancer 2001;84(2):199–201.

17. Mawrin C, Perry A. Pathological classification and molecular genetics of meningiomas. J Neurooncol 2010;99(3):379–91.

18. Gerber MA, Bahr SM, Gutmann DH. Protein 4.1B/ differentially expressed in adenocarcinoma of the lung-1 functions as a growth suppressor in meningioma cells by activating rac1-dependent c-Jun-NH(2)-kinase signaling. Cancer Res 2006;66(10): 5295–303.

19. Mawrin C, Sasse T, Kirches E, et al. Different activation of mitogen-activated protein kinase and Akt signaling is associated with aggressive phenotype of human meningiomas. Clin Cancer Res 2005;11(11):4074–82.

20. Brastianos PK, Horowitz PM, Santagata S, et al. Genomic sequencing of meningiomas identifies oncogenic SMO and AKT1 mutations. Nat Genet 2013;45(3):285–9.

21. Sami A, Karsy M. Targeting the PI3K/AKT/mTOR signaling pathway in glioblastoma: novel therapeutic agents and advances in understanding. Tumour Biol 2013;34(4):1991–2002.

22. Ragel BT, Jensen RL. Aberrant signaling pathways in meningiomas. J Neurooncol 2010;99(3): 315–24.

23. Santarpia L, Lippman SM, El-Naggar AK. Targeting the MAPK-RAS-RAF signaling pathway in cancer therapy. Expert Opin Ther Targets 2012;16(1): 103–19.

24. Johnson MD, Shaw AK, O'Connell MJ, et al. Analysis of transforming growth factor β receptor expression and signaling in higher grade meningiomas. J Neurooncol 2011;103(2):277–85.

25. Yaswen P, MacKenzie KL, Keith WN, et al. Therapeutic targeting of replicative immortality. Semin Cancer Biol 2015;35(Suppl):S104–28.

26. Bostrom J, Meyer-Puttlitz B, Wolter M, et al. Alterations of the tumor suppressor genes CDKN2A (p16(INK4a)), p14(ARF), CDKN2B (p15(INK4b)), and CDKN2C (p18(INK4c)) in atypical and anaplastic meningiomas. Am J Pathol 2001; 159(2):661–9.

27. Asghar U, Witkiewicz AK, Turner NC, et al. The history and future of targeting cyclin-dependent kinases in cancer therapy. Nat Rev Drug Discov 2015;14(2):130–46.

28. Laurendeau I, Ferrer M, Garrido D, et al. Gene expression profiling of the hedgehog signaling pathway in human meningiomas. Mol Med 2010; 16(7–8):262–70.

29. Baia GS, Stifani S, Kimura ET, et al. Notch activation is associated with tetraploidy and enhanced chromosomal instability in meningiomas. Neoplasia 2008;10(6):604–12.

30. Pecina-Slaus N, Nikuseva Martic T, Deak AJ, et al. Genetic and protein changes of E-cadherin in meningiomas. J Cancer Res Clin Oncol 2010;136(5): 695–702.

31. Clark VE, Erson-Omay EZ, Serin A, et al. Genomic analysis of non-NF2 meningiomas reveals mutations in TRAF7, KLF4, AKT1, and SMO. Science 2013;339(6123):1077–80.

32. Senol O, Schaaij-Visser TB, Erkan EP, et al. miR-200a-mediated suppression of non-muscle heavy chain IIb inhibits meningioma cell migration and tumor growth in vivo. Oncogene 2015;34(14): 1790–8.

33. Wang M, Deng X, Ying Q, et al. MicroRNA-224 targets ERG2 and contributes to malignant progressions of meningioma. Biochem Biophys Res Commun 2015;460(2):354–61.

34. Ludwig N, Kim YJ, Mueller SC, et al. Posttranscriptional deregulation of signaling pathways in meningioma subtypes by differential expression of miRNAs. Neuro Oncol 2015;17(9):1250–60.

35. Samoto K, Ikezaki K, Ono M, et al. Expression of vascular endothelial growth factor and its possible relation with neovascularization in human brain tumors. Cancer Res 1995;55(5):1189–93.

36. Dharmalingam P, Roopesh Kumar VR, Verma SK. Vascular endothelial growth factor expression and angiogenesis in various grades and subtypes of meningioma. Indian J Pathol Microbiol 2013; 56(4):349–54.

37. Lamszus K, Lengler U, Schmidt NO, et al. Vascular endothelial growth factor, hepatocyte growth factor/scatter factor, basic fibroblast growth factor, and placenta growth factor in human meningiomas and their relation to angiogenesis and malignancy. Neurosurgery 2000;46(4):938–47 [discussion: 947–8].

38. Wu Y, Lucia K, Lange M, et al. Hypoxia inducible factor-1 is involved in growth factor, glucocorticoid and hypoxia mediated regulation of vascular endothelial growth factor-A in human meningiomas. J Neurooncol 2014;119(2):263–73.

39. Wang P, Ni RY, Chen MN, et al. Expression of aquaporin-4 in human supratentorial meningiomas with peritumoral brain edema and correlation of VEGF with edema formation. Genet Mol Res 2011;10(3):2165–71.

40. Matuschek C, Bolke E, Nawatny J, et al. Bevacizumab as a treatment option for radiation-induced cerebral necrosis. Strahlenther Onkol 2011; 187(2):135–9.

41. Puchner MJ, Hans VH, Harati A, et al. Bevacizumab-induced regression of anaplastic meningioma. Ann Oncol 2010;21(12):2445–6.

42. Goutagny S, Raymond E, Sterkers O, et al. Radiographic regression of cranial meningioma in a NF2 patient treated by bevacizumab. Ann Oncol 2011; 22(4):990–1.

43. Wilson TJ, Heth JA. Regression of a meningioma during paclitaxel and bevacizumab therapy for breast cancer. J Clin Neurosci 2012;19(3):468–9.

44. Lou E, Sumrall AL, Turner S, et al. Bevacizumab therapy for adults with recurrent/progressive

meningioma: a retrospective series. J Neurooncol 2012;109(1):63–70.

45. Nayak L, Iwamoto FM, Rudnick JD, et al. Atypical and anaplastic meningiomas treated with bevacizumab. J Neurooncol 2012;109(1):187–93.

46. Hawasli AH, Rubin JB, Tran DD, et al. Antiangiogenic agents for nonmalignant brain tumors. J Neurol Surg B Skull Base 2013;74(3):136–41.

47. Nunes FP, Merker VL, Jennings D, et al. Bevacizumab treatment for meningiomas in NF2: a retrospective analysis of 15 patients. PLoS One 2013;8(3):e59941.

48. Raizer JJ, Grimm SA, Rademaker A, et al. A phase II trial of PTK787/ZK 222584 in recurrent or progressive radiation and surgery refractory meningiomas. J Neurooncol 2014;117(1):93–101.

49. Wen PY, Yung WK, Lamborn KR, et al. Phase II study of imatinib mesylate for recurrent meningiomas (North American Brain Tumor Consortium study 01-08). Neuro Oncol 2009;11(6):853–60.

50. Raizer JJ, Abrey LE, Lassman AB, et al. A phase I trial of erlotinib in patients with nonprogressive glioblastoma multiforme postradiation therapy, and recurrent malignant gliomas and meningiomas. Neuro Oncol 2010;12(1):87–94.

51. Norden AD, Raizer JJ, Abrey LE, et al. Phase II trials of erlotinib or gefitinib in patients with recurrent meningioma. J Neurooncol 2010;96(2):211–7.

52. Schrell UM, Rittig MG, Anders M, et al. Hydroxyurea for treatment of unresectable and recurrent meningiomas. II. Decrease in the size of meningiomas in patients treated with hydroxyurea. J Neurosurg 1997;86(5):840–4.

53. Newton HB, Slivka MA, Stevens C. Hydroxyurea chemotherapy for unresectable or residual meningioma. J Neurooncol 2000;49(2):165–70.

54. Mason WP, Gentili F, Macdonald DR, et al. Stabilization of disease progression by hydroxyurea in patients with recurrent or unresectable meningioma. J Neurosurg 2002;97(2):341–6.

55. Rosenthal MA, Ashley DL, Cher L. Treatment of high risk or recurrent meningiomas with hydroxyurea. J Clin Neurosci 2002;9(2):156–8.

56. Loven D, Hardoff R, Sever ZB, et al. Non-resectable slow-growing meningiomas treated by hydroxyurea. J Neurooncol 2004;67(1–2):221–6.

57. Hahn BM, Schrell UM, Sauer R, et al. Prolonged oral hydroxyurea and concurrent 3D-conformal radiation in patients with progressive or recurrent meningioma: results of a pilot study. J Neurooncol 2005;74(2):157–65.

58. Weston GJ, Martin AJ, Mufti GJ, et al. Hydroxyurea treatment of meningiomas: a pilot study. Skull Base 2006;16(3):157–60.

59. Chamberlain MC, Johnston SK. Hydroxyurea for recurrent surgery and radiation refractory meningioma: a retrospective case series. J Neurooncol 2011;104(3):765–71.

60. Chamberlain MC. Hydroxyurea for recurrent surgery and radiation refractory high-grade meningioma. J Neurooncol 2012;107(2):315–21.

61. Reardon DA, Norden AD, Desjardins A, et al. Phase II study of Gleevec(R) plus hydroxyurea (HU) in adults with progressive or recurrent meningioma. J Neurooncol 2012;106(2):409–15.

62. Kim MS, Yu DW, Jung YJ, et al. Long-term follow-up result of hydroxyurea chemotherapy for recurrent meningiomas. J Korean Neurosurg Soc 2012; 52(6):517–22.

63. Ragel BT, Gillespie DL, Kushnir V, et al. Calcium channel antagonists augment hydroxyurea- and RU486-induced inhibition of meningioma growth in vivo and in vitro. Neurosurgery 2006;59(5): 1109–20 [discussion: 1120–1].

64. Ragel BT, Couldwell WT, Wurster RD, et al. Chronic suppressive therapy with calcium channel antagonists for refractory meningiomas. Neurosurg Focus 2007;23(4):E10.

65. Jensen RL, Petr M, Wurster RD. Calcium channel antagonist effect on in vitro meningioma signal transduction pathways after growth factor stimulation. Neurosurgery 2000;46(3):692–702 [discussion: 702–3].

66. Grunberg SM, Daniels AM, Muensch H, et al. Correlation of meningioma hormone receptor status with hormone sensitivity in a tumor stem-cell assay. J Neurosurg 1987;66(3):405–8.

67. Grunberg SM, Weiss MH. Lack of efficacy of megestrol acetate in the treatment of unresectable meningioma. J Neurooncol 1990;8(1):61–5.

68. Jaaskelainen J, Laasonen E, Karkkainen J, et al. Hormone treatment of meningiomas: lack of response to medroxyprogesterone acetate (MPA). A pilot study of five cases. Acta Neurochir (Wien) 1986;80(1–2):35–41.

69. Grunberg SM, Weiss MH, Spitz IM, et al. Treatment of unresectable meningiomas with the antiprogesterone agent mifepristone. J Neurosurg 1991; 74(6):861–6.

70. Grunberg SM, Weiss MH, Russell CA, et al. Long-term administration of mifepristone (RU486): clinical tolerance during extended treatment of meningioma. Cancer Invest 2006;24(8):727–33.

71. Touat M, Lombardi G, Farina P, et al. Successful treatment of multiple intracranial meningiomas with the antiprogesterone receptor agent mifepristone (RU486). Acta Neurochir (Wien) 2014; 156(10):1831–5.

72. Lamberts SW, Tanghe HL, Avezaat CJ, et al. Mifepristone (RU 486) treatment of meningiomas. J Neurol Neurosurg Psychiatry 1992;55(6):486–90.

73. de Keizer RJ, Smit JW. Mifepristone treatment in patients with surgically incurable sphenoid-ridge meningioma: a long-term follow-up. Eye (Lond) 2004;18(9):954–8.

74. Cossu G, Levivier M, Daniel RT, et al. The role of mifepristone in meningiomas management: a systematic review of the literature. Biomed Res Int 2015;2015:267831.

75. Markwalder TM, Seiler RW, Zava DT. Antiestrogenic therapy of meningiomas–a pilot study. Surg Neurol 1985;24(3):245–9.

76. Goodwin JW, Crowley J, Eyre HJ, et al. A phase II evaluation of tamoxifen in unresectable or refractory meningiomas: a Southwest Oncology Group study. J Neurooncol 1993;15(1):75–7.

77. Ji J, Sundquist J, Sundquist K. Association of tamoxifen with meningioma: a population-based study in Sweden. Eur J Cancer Prev 2016;25(1): 29–33.

78. Chamberlain MC. Adjuvant combined modality therapy for malignant meningiomas. J Neurosurg 1996;84(5):733–6.

79. Chamberlain MC, Tsao-Wei DD, Groshen S. Temozolomide for treatment-resistant recurrent meningioma. Neurology 2004;62(7):1210–2.

80. Chamberlain MC, Tsao-Wei DD, Groshen S. Salvage chemotherapy with CPT-11 for recurrent meningioma. J Neurooncol 2006;78(3):271–6.

81. Gupta V, Su YS, Samuelson CG, et al. Irinotecan: a potential new chemotherapeutic agent for atypical or malignant meningiomas. J Neurosurg 2007; 106(3):455–62.

82. Preusser M, Spiegl-Kreinecker S, Lotsch D, et al. Trabectedin has promising antineoplastic activity in high-grade meningioma. Cancer 2012;118(20): 5038–49.

83. Balik V, Sulla I, Park HH, et al. In vitro testing to a panel of potential chemotherapeutics and current concepts of chemotherapy in benign meningiomas. Surg Oncol 2015;24(3):292–9.

84. Runzi MW, Jaspers C, Windeck R, et al. Successful treatment of meningioma with octreotide. Lancet 1989;1(8646):1074.

85. Garcia-Luna PP, Relimpio F, Pumar A, et al. Clinical use of octreotide in unresectable meningiomas. A report of three cases. J Neurosurg Sci 1993; 37(4):237–41.

86. Jaffrain-Rea ML, Minniti G, Santoro A, et al. Visual improvement during octreotide therapy in a case of episellar meningioma. Clin Neurol Neurosurg 1998;100(1):40–3.

87. Johnson DR, Kimmel DW, Burch PA, et al. Phase II study of subcutaneous octreotide in adults with recurrent or progressive meningioma and meningeal hemangiopericytoma. Neuro Oncol 2011; 13(5):530–5.

88. Simo M, Argyriou AA, Macia M, et al. Recurrent high-grade meningioma: a phase II trial with somatostatin analogue therapy. Cancer Chemother Pharmacol 2014;73(5):919–23.

89. Norden AD, Ligon KL, Hammond SN, et al. Phase II study of monthly pasireotide LAR (SOM230C) for recurrent or progressive meningioma. Neurology 2015;84(3):280–6.

90. Graillon T, Defilles C, Mohamed A, et al. Combined treatment by octreotide and everolimus: octreotide enhances inhibitory effect of everolimus in aggressive meningiomas. J Neurooncol 2015;124(1):33–43.

91. Kaba SE, DeMonte F, Bruner JM, et al. The treatment of recurrent unresectable and malignant meningiomas with interferon alpha-2B. Neurosurgery 1997;40(2):271–5.

92. Muhr C, Gudjonsson O, Lilja A, et al. Meningioma treated with interferon-alpha, evaluated with [(11) C]-L-methionine positron emission tomography. Clin Cancer Res 2001;7(8):2269–76.

93. Chamberlain MC. IFN-α for recurrent surgery- and radiation-refractory high-grade meningioma: a retrospective case series. CNS Oncol 2013;2(3): 227–35.

94. Friend KE, Radinsky R, McCutcheon IE. Growth hormone receptor expression and function in meningiomas: effect of a specific receptor antagonist. J Neurosurg 1999;91(1):93–9.

95. McCutcheon IE, Flyvbjerg A, Hill H, et al. Antitumor activity of the growth hormone receptor antagonist pegvisomant against human meningiomas in nude mice. J Neurosurg 2001;94(3):487–92.

96. Chiou HY, Lai WK, Huang LC, et al. Valproic acid promotes radiosensitization in meningioma stem-like cells. Oncotarget 2015;6(12):9959–69.

97. Koschny R, Boehm C, Sprick MR, et al. Bortezomib sensitizes primary meningioma cells to TRAIL-induced apoptosis by enhancing formation of the death-inducing signaling complex. J Neuropathol Exp Neurol 2014;73(11):1034–46.

98. El-Khatib M, Tepe C, Senger B, et al. Aminolevulinic acid-mediated photodynamic therapy of human meningioma: an in vitro study on primary cell lines. Int J Mol Sci 2015;16(5):9936–48.

99. Topalian SL, Sznol M, McDermott DF, et al. Survival, durable tumor remission, and long-term safety in patients with advanced melanoma receiving nivolumab. J Clin Oncol 2014;32(10):1020–30.

100. Brahmer JR, Tykodi SS, Chow LQ, et al. Safety and activity of anti-PD-L1 antibody in patients with advanced cancer. N Engl J Med 2012;366(26): 2455–65.

101. Du Z, Abedalthagafi M, Aizer AA, et al. Increased expression of the immune modulatory molecule PD-L1 (CD274) in anaplastic meningioma. Oncotarget 2015;6(7):4704–16.

Index

Note: Page numbers of article titles are in **boldface** type.

Neurosurg Clin N Am 27 (2016) 261–264
http://dx.doi.org/10.1016/S1042-3680(16)00017-6
1042-3680/16/$ – see front matter © 2016 Elsevier Inc. All rights reserved.

Moving?

Make sure your subscription moves with you!

To notify us of your new address, find your **Clinics Account Number** (located on your mailing label above your name), and contact customer service at:

Email: journalscustomerservice-usa@elsevier.com

800-654-2452 (subscribers in the U.S. & Canada)
314-447-8871 (subscribers outside of the U.S. & Canada)

Fax number: 314-447-8029

Elsevier Health Sciences Division
Subscription Customer Service
3251 Riverport Lane
Maryland Heights, MO 63043

ELSEVIER

Printed and bound by CPI Group (UK) Ltd, Croydon, CR0 4YY

08/05/2025

01864682-0004